MW00619871

Out with the OLD, **in with the NEW**

# spoiled milk

## 37 OLD Expired Health Beliefs **with a Fresh NEW Perspective**

Dr. Angela **Young**

Spoiled Milk: 37 OLD Expired Health Beliefs with a Fresh NEW Perspective


Print ISBN 978-1-61206-052-1



Cover Design: Cari Campbell of Cari Campbell Design

Interior Book Design: Fusion Creative Works, www.fusioncw.com

Primary Editor: Kim Foster

To order books in large quantities, please e-mail alohapublishing@gmail.com or call 208-344-2733.

To contact Dr. Angela Young about speaking or consulting, contact Live Right Chiropractic at 208-383-3703.

Published by

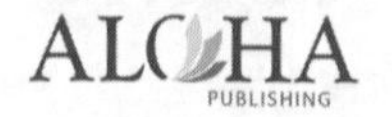


AlohaPublishing.com

Second Printing

Printed in the United States of America

# dedication

*For Janette, Sarah, Liz, and Gabby*

# contents

## Food 41

# about spoiled milk

If you ever get a whiff of spoiled milk, you won't like what you smell. It's not anything worth keeping. You can't drink it, and if you tried, you could get sick. Just as spoiled milk doesn't deserve a place in your fridge, there are many common health myths floating around that have absolutely no place in your life.

Spoiled Milk was written to expose the mind-sets and methods of 37 out-of-date, inaccurate beliefs that impact your health. Each chapter has a "Fresh Ideas to Extend Your Expiration Date" section with tips to help you reach your full health potential. Throw out those old-fashioned, outdated myths that are making you sick and reducing your quality of life, and feel good again!

Dr. Angela **Young**

# introduction

How do you know what to believe? Many common ideas of health are based on popular fads that are altogether false. Advertising, marketing, and self-interested research drive these fads. These theories may cost you time, money, and most importantly, your health. You need to reconsider the health myths that stifle your good health and prevent you from achieving your full health potential.

Many health concepts are learned intuitively. If a plant is sick or wilting, you know how to make its environment more hospitable for thriving: provide good soil, adequate sunlight, and enough water. It would be odd to consider giving it a pill or performing surgery on it. You would simply change the plant's environment. Change the environment and you can change the health of the plant. We often forget that health can be that simple.

*Spoiled Milk* was written to answer your common health questions, plus address those pervasive beliefs that are often encountered among friends, family, and patients in my chiropractic practice. This book encourages the development of new beliefs to change the American mind-set regarding health. Although the research is new, the concepts are timeless and are based on facts, solid research, and good, old-fashioned common sense.

We've been surviving on this planet for generations by following these rules—rules we weren't even aware of. The ideas in *Spoiled Milk* will get you excited about learning more about yourself, and, most importantly, finding ways to apply these fresh ideas to your life and the lives of your loved ones.

# Wellness

America is in a health crisis. Currently, it is struggling with instances of "lifestyle diseases" that are often preventable. Lifestyle diseases include atherosclerosis, heart disease, stroke, obesity, type 2 diabetes, and diseases associated with smoking, alcohol, and drug abuse.

Here is a look at causes of death in 2007 versus 1900.[1]

Main causes of death in 2007:

1. Heart disease
2. Cancer
3. Stroke
4. Chronic lower respiratory diseases
5. Accidents

Main causes of death in 1900:

1. Pneumonia, Influenza
2. Tuberculosis
3. GI disorders
4. Heart disease
5. Stroke

As you can see, there are huge differences between the causes of death in 1900, which were more commonly due to diseases that are now easily treatable, and causes of death in 2007, which are lifestyle related.

Current beliefs about health and wellness are not working. Health care costs are rising by the billions each year. More time, energy, and money are spent at doctor appointments, hospitals, labs, filling prescriptions, tests, and waiting for the results. Time is also spent making the money to pay for those things. Wouldn't you rather spend your time, energy, and money doing the things you love?

The entire way health is defined needs to be shifted. Beliefs about being healthy are always changing, such as sickness is an event versus a process and health is a gift of winning a genetic lottery. These beliefs are just not true. Changing the way you think about health is the first step in the process of getting healthy and staying healthy. Most health decisions are based on "losing belly fat" or losing weight. Getting trim may be an effect of getting healthy, but there are a lot of unhealthy ways to get there. True wellness is a journey, not a quick fix. The following are common wellness myths that shape what you believe.

# spoiler alert

*If you think being thin is all that matters,*

consider

*that your health is not determined by how much or how little you weigh.*

Getting skinny, burning fat, and losing weight are the purposes of eating right, exercise, and self-care. Although this seems to be the major media message blaring out, skinny doesn't equal healthy. You can lose weight and get thin by starving yourself, purging, taking pills, smoking, doing drugs, crash dieting, or experiencing a life-threatening disease. It may mean you look thin, but it doesn't make you healthy. Chemical substances can make you thin, and some people can stay skinny with a poor diet and no exercise. Eating nutrient-depleted, processed foods may cause you to lose weight, but it is not a recipe for building a healthy body because healthy and skinny do not equal the same thing.

The goal of this book is to help you get healthy, to feel good, and to have a good quality of life where you can do the things you want to do and enjoy your life. A lot of the time, healthy people are thin because they are active, eat well, and take good care of themselves. But don't confuse getting skinny with getting healthy. Risks of cardiovascular disease, diabetes, and obesity-related health problems do tend to decrease with weight loss, but skinny people can still be unhealthy. Thinking that getting healthy is synonymous with being thin and losing weight is like thinking that money will make you happy. They may go together, but it is not guaranteed.

> “*It's important to be healthy on the inside and on the outside. Some people can eat all kinds of junk and still stay slim, but that doesn't mean they're healthy.*”
>
> – Karen Ansel, spokeswoman from American Dietetic Association, *Shape Magazine*

## Fresh Ideas to Extend Your Expiration Date

1. The means are as important as the end. If your goal is to look good, lose weight, and get great abs, that is fine, but why not do it the healthy way?

2. Make a list of your health goals—what you want for now, six months from now, and one year from now. Getting skinny can be one of them, but you can be skinny and still feel bad. How do you want to feel and what do you want to be able to do when you feel good?

3. Realize that feeling good has less to do with how you look and more to do with how healthy your self-image is. Feeling good about yourself is attractive, no matter your size.

## Learn More

*America the Beautiful 2*, a documentary by Darryl Roberts, is an insightful look into the diet industry and whether it is possible to be healthy at a variety of weights.

spoiler alert

*If you think what is considered healthy is always changing,*

consider

*that we are being influenced by advertising hype and the interests of those doing the research.*

Research has its place and it is used in this book, but it is always helpful to answer these questions:

- *Who profits from me believing this?*
- *Who profits from this lotion, vitamin, diet, weight-loss strategy, pill, or surgery?*
- *Do they have my best interests at heart?*

Many health-seeking people are very confused about what is healthy because the research results are always changing. One day, Echinacea is proved to be the cure for everything. The next day, week, month, or year, it is proved to be the cure for nothing. One day carbohydrates are bad, and the next day they are preventing colon cancer. In with vitamin D…out with vitamin D.

A common question is, "How do I evaluate the mountain of health information that I read?" If you google "health," it will come up with thousands of different perspectives and different cures. Staying healthy is very unsensational and is based on easy guidelines.

> “*Everyone should be his own physician. We ought to assist and not force nature. Eat with moderation what agrees with your constitution. Nothing is good for the body but what we can digest. What medicine can produce digestion? Exercise. What will recruit strength? Sleep. What will alleviate incurable ills? Patience.*”
>
> – Voltaire

## Fresh Ideas to Extend Your Expiration Date

Ask these questions to determine what is healthy:

1. What are the lifestyle choices someone living at the turn of the 20th century would have made compared to the choices I am making now?

In terms of nutrition, they ate mostly fresh, unprocessed foods. Exercise was a part of their daily lifestyles. They also had reduced chemical and toxin exposure from their environment and the products they used.

2. What is the most natural choice, and am I making that choice?

3. Are my decisions based on hype and fads or on what is actually good for me?

4. Where is this info coming from and who benefits from me buying this supplement, vitamin, food, or exercise plan?

Long-term, sustainable health choices are very simple. They include the very things that make plants flourish and other mammals healthy: good food, clean environment and water, movement and activity, exposure to sunlight, and adequate rest. If you apply the concepts of what keeps the planet healthy to your own life, then fads are a thing of the past and healthy decisions are easy. Pick strategies to deal with stress, health, nutrition, and movement plans that are sustainable for a lifetime. This is a life plan, not a two-week vacation.

## Learn More

*The Blue Zones: Lessons for Living Longer from People Who've Lived the Longest*, by Dan Buettner, is a great book for health advice from centenarians from different cultures.

*The Blue Zones* blog includes articles, recipes and healthy tips at bluezones.com/blog.

This website contains quizzes to assess your vitality, determine your biological age versus healthy life expectancy based on your life habits, and includes suggestions for improvement: apps.bluezones.com/vitality.

# spoiler alert

***If you think you are sick because you aren't taking the right drug or haven't had the right surgery,***

**consider**

***that the real cause is often found at a deeper level.***

People are generally sick due to physical, emotional, and mental stresses, or environmental and chemical traumas and exposures. People are not getting sick because they are deficient in antibiotics, and they're not having heart attacks because they are deficient in open heart surgeries. There is also no such disease that causes a pain pill deficiency. People are sick because their bodies can no longer keep up with the demands placed on them, and something has got to give. Generally, that "something" results in an illness.

Symptoms are how the body lets you know what it needs. They are like flashing lights that you should pay attention to before you develop a chronic illness or pain. Hunger and thirst are symptoms, but that doesn't mean they are bad; they mean you need to eat and drink. Sleepiness is a symptom, but that doesn't mean it's something negative; it means you need to rest. Without these symptoms or feedback, you would not survive. You would starve, burn out from exhaustion, or die from dehydration.

Drugs and surgery do not address the physiology behind the chronic disease. They merely change the indicators of disease—they decrease blood glucose for diabetes and decrease lipid levels for high triglycerides. Arteries are mechanically cleared with surgery versus addressing why the arteries are clogged in the first place. Drugs and surgery will never be a fix for chronic health problems because they don't change what created the problem in the first place.

*"Drugs never cure disease. They merely hush the voice of nature's protest, and pull down the danger signals she erects along the pathway of transgression. Any poison taken into the system has to be reckoned with later on even though it palliates present symptoms. Pain may disappear, but the patient is left in a worse condition, though unconscious of it at the time."*

– Daniel H. Kress, MD

## Fresh Ideas to Extend Your Expiration Date

Learn to examine the real cause of pain and disease. It will change your mind-set when you have symptoms. For example, instead of reaching for a pain reliever for a headache as a short-term solution, determine to find the underlying cause. It may be a reaction to a smell you are sensitive to, hormonal fluctuations, something you ate or didn't eat, something you drank or didn't drink, muscle tension, stress, or something going on in your neck. It is not an aspirin, pain pill, or drug deficiency. Use this same system of evaluation before treating pain with "Band-Aid" cures, which are only masking a deeper problem.

This evaluation can be used for any symptom.

1. Acknowledge your symptoms and begin to think of your aches and pains as intelligent signals instead of something to be silenced.
2. Identify what may be the underlying cause of your symptoms.
3. Address the factors that may be contributing to the cause of your symptoms.
4. Prevent the factors or the environment that creates the symptom from even occurring. As Benjamin Franklin said, "an ounce of prevention is worth a pound of cure."

## Learn More

The website drhyman.com has an insightful blog that addresses the evaluation of symptoms. Check out the blog post titled "Why Treating Your Symptoms Is a Recipe for Disaster."

*Ultraprevention: The 6-Week Plan That Will Make You Healthy for Life*, by Dr. Mark Hyman and Mark Liponis, has an innovative look at what it really means to be well and what symptoms represent.

# spoiler alert

*If you think you have to be sick to get better,*

consider

*changing your definition of health.*

It is easy to limit the definition of health. To some, it is merely the absence of sickness, symptoms, or pain. But what is true health? The World Health Organization defines it as "a state of complete physical, mental, and social well-being and not merely the absence of disease or infirmity." Most people live just above the crisis line without sickness and symptoms but do not truly live well. You can always strive towards greater health and make healthy decisions for yourself, regardless if you feel sick.

Some diseases, such as viruses, have a rapid onset, but many diseases are chronic with a slow progression made possible by their environment. Researchers believe that some cancers take years to develop before they are detectable with current testing procedures. Your body is in a constant state of adaptation in response to your environment, shifting toward sickness or health at any time. Health is a continuum with disease on one end and good health on the other. You are in constant motion between the two, either shifting toward or away from health.

You can constantly be reaching for your higher health potential. Just like in exercise, you can always train yourself to run faster, swim farther, and jump higher. You can also reach greater levels of health by being proactive versus being reactive—consistently making healthy choices regardless of how you feel. Don't wait until you begin to feel bad, have symptoms, or experience a health crisis to make healthy changes.

> *"The physician who teaches people to sustain their health is the superior physician. The physician who waits to treat people until after their health is lost is considered to be inferior. This is like waiting until one's family is starving to begin to plant seeds in the garden."*
>
> – Ilza Veith and Ken Rose, *The Yellow Emperor's Classic of Internal Medicine*

## Fresh Ideas to Extend Your Expiration Date

Change your definition of health by making decisions with the end in mind. You wouldn't wait until your car runs out of gas to fill it up. That would be far more time consuming, dramatic, and would leave you stranded. Fill up your car while there is enough gas to get you to a fuel station. Don't wait until an emergency to make healthy choices.

Healthy choices consist of simple additions that will direct you toward health, even if you don't have any symptoms. Ask yourself, "What can I add to take my health to the next level?" Eventually you can begin to remove the unhealthy habits you have, but if you have already made healthy additions, it will be much easier.

- Add a fruit or veggie to your meal.
- Add an after-dinner walk.
- Add contemplation and meditation into your daily routine.
- Think about and act on a simple healthy addition you can make to your life.

Make the leap from surviving to thriving. Don't wait until a health crisis to search for a cure.

## Learn More

In *Revive: Stop Feeling Spent and Start Living Again*, Frank Lipman, MD, gives tips for integrating a wellness lifestyle into your life. His blog, located at drfranklipman.com, is full of helpful health strategies and video tips.

# spoiler alert

*If you think your genetic profile will determine your health,*

consider

*that your genes can either be turned on or off by lifestyle choices.*

For years, the medical profession held to the belief that everything was determined by genetic code. With only 25,000–35,000 genes in the human genome, scientists eventually discovered that there is no way this number of genes could represent the complexity of humans.

A developing field in the study of epigenetics shows how factors or environmental signals outside the genetic code determine gene expression or repression. The findings show that the environment regulates gene activity. Simply put, you may have genetic markers for autoimmune disorders, but your environmental inputs and choices determine what happens next. If you make unhealthy dietary and activity choices and do not have strategies in place to cope with stress, the autoimmune markers may be "turned on" and you will express symptoms. With healthy dietary and activity choices and high resilience to stress, the gene may be repressed and you will not display autoimmune symptoms. These findings put you in control of how your genes express themselves. You can't just blame or praise your genetics for your health or lack of it. Your genes are simply responding to environmental signals.

> "*When the cultured cells you are studying are ailing, you look first to the cell's environment, not to the cell itself, for the cause. When I provided a healthy environment for my cells, they thrived; when the environment was less than optimal, the cells faltered. When I adjusted the environment, these 'sick' cells revitalized.*"
>
> – Bruce Lipton, *The Biology of Belief: Unleashing the Power of Consciousness, Matter & Miracles*

## Fresh Ideas to Extend Your Expiration Date

Stop blaming your genes and start providing a healthy environment for your cells to thrive. Consider that your genes aren't making you sick, overweight, or out of shape. Your cells are responding to the environment.

Steps to make a healthy environment:

1. Your thoughts control how you respond to life. Stop blaming your "bad genes" for your health.
2. Six basic foundations for a healthy environment for your genes to healthily express themselves:
   - Sleep: Get six to eight hours a night.
   - Sun: Spend 20 minutes a day in the sun without sunscreen.
   - Movement and activity: Move more every day.
   - Healthy thoughts and engagement in life: Love the life you live and check the pipeline of negativity (the media, Facebook, TV, and Internet) that you consume.
   - Good nutrition: Include lots of fresh veggies, and if you eat animal products, choose well-raised animal products. Don't forget to include adequate hydration.
   - Chemicals: Limit your exposure to cleaning products, personal care products, alcohol, legal or illegal drugs, smoking, room fresheners, and sprays.

## Learn More

"Why Your DNA Isn't Your Destiny," by John Cloud, is an article that goes in-depth about the science behind epigenetics and is located at time.com.

*The Biology of Belief: Unleashing the Power of Consciousness, Matter & Miracles*, by Bruce Lipton, and *The Epigenetics Revolution: How Modern Biology is Rewriting Our Understanding of Genetics, Disease, and Inheritance*, by Nessa Carey, are two books that make epigenetics understandable.

# spoiler alert

***If you think your body is "broken" and cannot be repaired and pain is just a part of getting old,***

## consider

***that the body is created to heal.***

Your body is designed to be a self-healing system. When it receives a paper cut, if kept free of infection, it heals on its own without intervention. The body recognizes the cut and adapts to the situation and closes the wound—all without your help or instruction. The same body that heals a paper cut is able to heal torn muscles, fractures, broken bones, and torn ligaments, largely without intervention.

The self-healing intelligence that heals a paper cut can heal "bad" knees, hips, wrists, and elbows, given the right support. They aren't actually body parts that don't work; they have simply adapted to the stressors placed on them. The best thing you can do for your body is give it the ingredients it needs to self-heal and then get out of the way of the healing process. Aging is natural, but you don't have to age with pain and bad health. People say, "I have knee pain in my right knee because I was a runner, and now I am just getting old." The reality is both knees are the same age, so why doesn't the other one hurt? Pain and deterioration don't have to be normal or what you expect.

> “*Most of what we call aging is decay, and decay is optional: it's under our control.*”
>
> – Henry S. Lodge, MD, coauthor, *Younger Next Year: Live Strong, Fit, and Sexy—until You're 80 and Beyond*

## Fresh Ideas to Extend Your Expiration Date

Most people know surprisingly little about how their bodies work. Your body is what allows you to access the world. A key to wellness is tuning into how your body works on a day-to-day basis—appreciating all of the things it easily allows you to do. For most people, eating, breathing, walking, digesting, rebuilding, repairing, and blood circulating are done without much notice. It is amazing if you stop to think about it. Learning about and paying attention to what your body does may enhance a sense of gratefulness versus contempt or compassion for yourself because a body part is not working right.

Steps to allow healing:

1. Stop thinking you are "broken" or hurting because you are getting old. You become what you think.
2. Make choices that nourish your body's inborn ability to self-heal. These include good nutrition, good movement, good sleep, and good thoughts.
3. Instead of using the label of "bad" to describe something, consider that you have an area that is in the process of healing and needs some attention.

## Learn More

A best-selling, interesting look at aging versus decay and what you can do about it is *Younger Next Year: Live Strong, Fit, and Sexy—until You're 80 and Beyond*, by Chris Crowley and Henry S. Lodge, MD. This one is geared toward men, but they also wrote *Younger Next Year for Women: Live Strong, Fit, and Sexy—until You're 80 and Beyond.*

> “*We overlook the reality that most of us are healthy most of the time, the reality that the human organism has remarkable self-healing capacities for adaption and survival.*”
>
> – Arthur J. Basky, *Worried Sick, Our Troubled Quest for Wellness*

# Food

Food is one of the most misunderstood facets of health. It is necessary for your survival. In other health books, this section could have easily been labeled "Nutrition." However, this makes nutrients and food seem separate from each other, causing you to focus on eating certain nutrients without looking at the food as a whole. Although you ingest nutrients when you eat food, fundamentally you eat food, not nutrients. This distinction is important and may be what has contributed to some of the confusion about food. You have to look at food as a whole; a vegetable is more than the sum of its nutrient parts.

This section will address your health woes, fears, and common misconceptions where food is concerned. Choosing what to eat is often made to be complicated, and the rules about it seem very confusing. There is a lot of unhealthy food masquerading as healthy food. With a myriad of health choices, how do you pick what is right for you?

It doesn't have to be difficult. The simplest answer is to eat real food. But what is real food? It is traditional food that has been eaten since the beginning of time, not chemicals impersonating real food. Traditional food is food you can make in your kitchen. It does not need to be concocted in a lab of food scientists. It is grown from the earth or comes from animals. This means, instead of eating Pop-tarts, crackers shaped like goldfish, or potato chips that taste like a loaded baked potato, you eat food that you can make yourself.

A good rule to follow is if you can't make it without a team of flavoring specialists, don't eat it. Before you put something in your mouth, ask yourself, "what is the most traditional, natural form of this food?" Wasabi-encrusted peas or peas from the garden? Sugar-covered breakfast cereals, chips, soda, and flavored crystals that dissolve in water are hardly traditional or natural. These are food-like substances that preceding generations would not know what to think of. How close to traditional and unprocessed can you get? Whole milk versus skim milk; whole mozzarella versus fat-free mozzarella; fresh or frozen peas versus canned peas. Pick the food that is closest to how it exists in nature.

# spoiler alert

*If you think the fat/carbohydrate/protein label on food is the determinant of health,*

consider

*buying real foods without a label.*

Most people assume that it is the proportion of fat, carbs, and proteins that makes a food healthy rather than the actual ingredients. Michael Pollan dubbed this as the "Science of Nutritionism" in *Defense of Food: An Eater's Manifesto*. The ingredients may be all chemicals, taste enhancers, artificial additives, or things known to contribute to inflammation. You can get a balanced meal based on government recommendations from your favorite fast food chain, but that doesn't mean it is of good quality.

There are three major problems with the theory that health can be determined by the fat/carbohydrate/protein ratio:

1. It does not take into account the quality or components of the food. It may be full of hydrolyzed proteins, trans fats, chemicals, preservatives, dyes, artificial flavors, and sweeteners. However, based on the fat, carbohydrate, or protein content, it may still be deemed healthy and labeled as an important part of a balanced diet.

2. Researchers are still figuring out all the things that make whole foods (fruits and veggies) nutritionally beneficial. They know there are carbs, proteins, fats, vitamins, and minerals. But what about the antioxidants, flavonoids, phenols, and carotenoids? It is difficult to create foods in a lab that are as nutritious as foods nature grows when all of what makes it nutritious has not been identified.

3. What is considered to be good for you often changes: currently protein is in and carbs and fat are out.

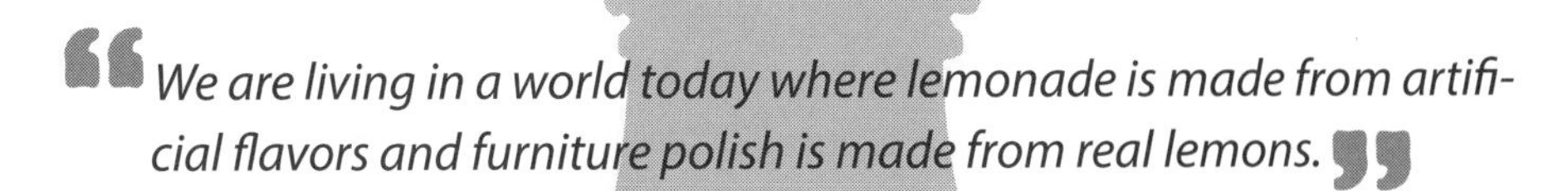

> *We are living in a world today where lemonade is made from artificial flavors and furniture polish is made from real lemons.*
>
> – Alfred E. Newman

## Fresh Ideas to Extend Your Expiration Date

Change your mind-set about what a healthy food actually is by focusing on the ingredients versus the narrow view of the fat/carbohydrate/protein ratio. The real concern should be the ingredients that are making up the food.

1. Eliminate ingredients you can't pronounce.

2. Eliminate ingredients that you aren't able to purchase separately or have never heard of before.

3. Eat whole foods that don't have ingredient labels, such as apples, carrots, celery, and many more primarily located in the periphery of the grocery store or at your local farmer's market. Real foods, such as fruits and vegetables, don't need ingredient labels.

4. Double check products you assume are healthy based on marketing or packaging. For example, look at the so-called healthy exercise bars

and sports drinks loaded with chemicals, additives, and sugars. Even though they have a healthy fat/carbohydrate/protein ratio, they are full of other bad-for-you ingredients. Better yet, don't buy them at all. Substitute a banana with almond butter for your after-workout snack, and skip the labels and the harmful ingredients all together.

As the old adage goes, "An apple a day keeps the doctor away." Note it does not say the apple-flavored Pop-tart or the apple-flavored cereal.

## Learn More

A blog with extensive recipes for families is located at 100daysofrealfood.com. It started as a project to eat whole foods on a budget with a family of four and has turned into a wildly popular blog on "real" food.

Download the Whole Foods app for your smart phone or tablet. It's a magical app that is easy to use with a lot of great recipes using real food.

*In Defense of Food: An Eater's Manifesto,* by Michael Pollan, is a simple, clear approach to food written by a journalist and is an excellent resource for making real food choices. *Food Rules: An Eater's Manual*, by the same author, is a small, easily readable book that makes food choices easy and entertaining.

# spoiler alert

*If you think a low-fat or no-fat diet keeps you skinny and healthy,*

consider

*that it may actually help put on the weight.*

When people recount their diets, they commonly claim, "I try to eat low fat." This is seen as a virtue but is based on poor research. Fat has a bad reputation. Sadly, it is the villain of the fat/carbohydrate/protein triad.

When you take all the fats out of your diet, you eat more carbohydrates to replace them. Increased carbohydrates raise your blood sugar and insulin levels without making you feel full like fat does. Fat stimulates the feel-full hormone, CCK. Increased carbohydrate intake, especially fructose, has been linked to the rise in obesity and type 2 diabetes. Excess cholesterol may also be produced by eating a high-carbohydrate diet.

Saturated fat has been implicated in causing heart disease, so decreasing it is supposed to decrease the risk of heart disease. This is only partially true. Decreasing saturated fats from hydrogenated vegetable oils (such as shortening) decreases the risk of heart disease. Decreasing saturated fats altogether may not decrease the risk like once thought.

Many vegetables have fat-soluble nutrients in them, which means they are absorbed better when eaten with a fat. Focus on keeping a high level of Omega-3 fatty acids (important for decreasing inflammation) as compared to Omega-6 fatty acids (which can contribute to causing inflammation). Long-term inflammation has been linked to multiple diseases, including cancer, arthritis, heart disease, and chronic pain. Focus on healthy fats and only eat organic or pastured meats, which are high in Omega-3.

> *It is now increasingly recognized that the low-fat campaign has been based on little scientific evidence and may have caused unintended health problems.*
>
> – Dr. Hu, *Journal of the American College of Nutrition*

## Fresh Ideas to Extend Your Expiration Date

Buy full-fat products. Lite, no-fat, and low-fat products have added sugar and chemicals to make them taste good and give them a more compelling texture. Eat foods with real fat, not processed fake fat. There is processed fat in cookies, chips, salad dressings, and margarine.

Check out the appendix for tables with healthy fat guidelines.

Not all fats are good, mind you. Fats that aren't good include trans fats commonly found in margarines, chips, and processed foods. Trans fats are still around. Even when labeled "no trans fats," it is not always true. It just means there is less than .5 percent per serving. Trans fats are proven to lead to heart disease and inflammation. It's confusing because most health experts focus on low fat. You have to completely flip your mind-set. Eat your egg yolks. Don't be scared of the fat in organic meat. Embrace it and learn to eat it.

## Learn More

*Real Food: What to Eat and Why*, by Nina Planck, is an easily readable book about the benefits of real foods and real fats. She presents relatable, straightforward, and easily implementable ideas garnished with research and common sense.

Gary Taubes is the author of two books, *Why We Get Fat: And What to Do about It* and *Good Calories, Bad Calories: Fat, Carbs, and the Controversial Science of Diet and Health*. These books contain research supporting the hypothesis that consuming fat does not contribute to weight gain. His website, garytaubes.com, is a wealth of information with links to the various articles he has written on this subject.

# spoiler alert

***If you think the only difference between organic and inorganic food products is the price,***

## consider

***that organic foods have less pesticides and higher Omega-3 content.***

The jury is still out on organic versus inorganic food. A multitude of research shows support for both sides. A widely publicized, 2012 Stanford University meta-analysis of 250 studies came to the conclusion that "it did not find strong evidence that organic foods were more nutritious or carry fewer health risks than conventional alternatives."[1]

However, researchers did find that organic food has more phenols, which are linked to antioxidant activity. This protects your DNA from damage. Organic eggs and chickens contain more Omega-3 (an anti-inflammatory, essential fatty acid), there is 30 percent less pesticide residue on organic produce, and chicken and pork contain less antibiotic-resistant bacteria. These good things translate into a difference, unlike the study claims.

A huge difference between organic and inorganic is genetically modified organisms (GMO), super plants with increased yields and a built-in resistance to insects and pests. Unfortunately, these super plants have downsides, including links to infertility,[2] organ failure,[3] and cancer.[4] They are not required to be labeled in the United States, so unless you're eating organic, you may be eating GMOs.

Organic animal products contain less hormones, antibiotics, and toxins, and contain more of what makes animals healthy to eat. Genetically modified, pesticide-covered feeds, unnatural feedlot lifestyles, increased antibiotics, and growth hormones are all passed along to the consumer. If an animal is raised unhealthily and you consume the animal, how does that make you healthy? The health of the animal becomes your health also.

*High-tech tomatoes. Mysterious milk. Supersquash. Are we supposed to eat this stuff? Or is it going to eat us?*

– Annita Manning

## Fresh Ideas to Extend Your Expiration Date

To my knowledge, there are no studies showing that conventional farming is better or superior to the organic approach. Evaluate the inorganic versus organic question by what is more natural or more capable of producing health. Ingesting pesticides, herbicides, and chemical fertilizers could be harmful to your health. They are obviously sprayed on and around the plants, affecting both the plants and the soil quality. Organic is the best choice to decrease exposure to pesticides, herbicides, and GMO products.

If you have to decide between organic produce and organic animal products, pick organic animal products. Organic animal products are a far superior product to their nonorganic counterparts. For example, nonorganic cows are mostly fed a diet of GMO corn and soy, which they are not designed to eat. They are designed to eat grasses. Due to high corn prices in 2012, cows were being fed candy as it was cheaper than their regular feed. Candy to cows? That can't possibly make them healthy. Oftentimes these unnatural diets make them sick, causing an increase in antibiotic use. To top it off, growth hormones are often added to increase production.

Inorganic produce is designated with a barcode that starts with a 4 (for example, 4232). Organic starts with a 9. Be aware that organic cookies, crackers, and cereal may be marginally better than their nonorganic equals because of no GMOs or pesticides, but they still aren't the best choice.

## Learn More

*To Buy or Not to Buy Organic: What You Need to Know to Choose the Healthiest, Safest, Most Earth-Friendly Food*, by Cindy Burke, is a very practical organic guide to food. If you have an unlimited budget, always eat organic. If you have to pick and choose, this is the book for you.

*Organic Manifesto: How Organic Farming Can Heal Our Planet, Feed the World, and Keep Us Safe,* by Maria Rodale, is a very slanted view towards organic food as the name suggests. She provides a very readable synopsis of how organic is good for the planet as a whole, versus just for us as individual eaters.

Can't find grass-fed meats in your area? Go to eatwild.com to find local farmers in your area, or check out grasslandbeef.com and grassfedorganics.com for good meat sources you can have delivered to your door.

For a complete list of the dirty dozen and clean 15 foods, visit ewg.org/foodnews.

# spoiler alert

***If you think diet or zero-calorie foods and drinks will help you cut calories,***

consider

***that they could be causing weight gain and damaging your health.***

Zero calories. Sounds tempting right? In the dangerous pursuit to get thin, people are doing more harm than good. In the effort to reduce calories, they buy diet drinks, lite juices, and lite desserts. These may reduce sugar content, but they increase chemical intake. NutraSweet, Equal, Sweet'N Low, and Splenda (supposedly "natural" but produced by chlorinating a sucrose molecule), and neotame are all names of the most popular artificial sweeteners.

If you avoid products with labels, then you generally don't have to worry about these chemicals. Diet sodas have been linked to an increase in heart disease, stroke, risk of type 2 diabetes, occurrences of bladder cancer, and kidney damage. Plus, they have been linked to weight gain instead of weight loss! It is possibly because artificially sweetened beverages stimulate your brain, causing the desire to ingest sweets.[5]

Artificial sweeteners may be FDA approved, but that doesn't make them safe. The body does not metabolize them for energy. They supposedly pass through the digestive tract unassimilated and unprocessed. The body is created to respond to its environment. It is hard to imagine that an unnatural, artificial substance could enter the body without the body's defenses reacting.

These chemicals do not naturally occur anywhere else and are linked to an abundance of health issues. One may argue that chemicals don't hurt. However, do they really help? Maybe the question shouldn't be, do they make you sick? Maybe it should be, do they make you healthier?

> *As I see it, every day you do one of two things: build health or produce disease in yourself.*
>
> – Adelle Davis

## Fresh Ideas to Extend Your Expiration Date

Avoid sugar-free, "diet," no-added sugar, zero-calorie, cookies, ice creams, juices, desserts, and jams. Stay away from making recipes that call for artificial sweeteners. Artificial sweeteners are packaged under many different names: sucralose, Splenda, aspartame, neotame, NutraSweet, Equal, Sweet'N Low, saccharin, Sweet Twin, Necta Sweet, acesulfame-K, Sunett, and Sweet One. In moderation, stevia is the best noncaloric sweetener. You can even grow it yourself!

Skip the diet beverages. Water is the best no-calorie beverage to drink. Need more flavor? Water made at home, infused with essential oils or real lemon, lime, and mint, is tasty, real, and has health benefits. Herbal teas and Metromint water are also great no-additive drinks. Having been artificial sweetener free for three years, I can instantly taste them in beverages and sweets. They have a distinct, extremely sweet, fake flavor. The less fake sweeteners you consume, the more you notice when they are the sweetener choice in a product or recipe.

## Learn More

Two documentaries that show a different side to artificial sweeteners are *Sweet Misery: A Poisoned World* and *Sweet Remedy: The World Reacts to an Adulterated Food Supply*. Both of these can be watched for free online at youtube.com.

Russell Blaylock's book, *Excitotoxins: The Taste That Kills*, looks at the potential effects of artificial sweeteners and other chemical additives.

# spoiler alert

*If you think soy is a health food,*

consider

*the hormonal effects it may have on the body.*

Soy has gained popularity in the United States as a health food, and it is increasingly available in almost every processed food. It is hyped as a health food because the Japanese and Chinese eat it and tend to have longer life spans than Americans. However, this is not the whole story.

Eighty to 90 percent of soy is genetically modified. It is hard to digest, causes stomach upsets, and it can depress thyroid function and increase estrogen levels.[6] This can lead to estrogen dominance, which is bad in both men and women and may contribute to certain types of cancer. Two glasses of soy milk a day have enough hormones to alter a woman's menstrual cycle. It is high in Omega-6 fatty acids as well, which has been proven to be inflammatory.

Soy is commonly used because it is an inexpensive protein, and it increases the shelf life of processed foods. The only types of soy you should consume are fermented types of soy, which include natto, tempeh, and miso. The soy that is available in processed foods (soy oil, vegetable oil, edamame, most soy sauces, and tofu) is unfermented. The fermentation process deactivates or lessens the effects of the enzyme inhibitors (which make it harder to digest) and phytates (which block the absorption of important minerals in your body) in the soy.

> "*I'm still a bit cautious about soy, especially about eating a lot of it. Soy may have a dark side.*"
>
> – Walter C. Willet, MD, *Eat, Drink, and Be Healthy: The Harvard Medical School Guide to Healthy Eating*

## Fresh Ideas to Extend Your Expiration Date

Soy should be avoided unless it has been fermented, but this is difficult when buying processed foods. If you can't avoid soy, at least buy organic because organic is not genetically modified.

Tips for avoiding soy:

1. Avoid any type of nonfermented soy, including, but not limited to, edamame, soy sauce, tofu, soy oils, and hydrolyzed soy protein. Watch out for soy, which is often found in most processed foods, vegetable oils, infant formula, dressings, ice creams, sauces, breads, and protein powders.

2. If you are going to buy food with labels, then become an avid label reader. It is possible to find food without soy in them. It may take longer at first, but the benefits of health far outweigh the time cost.

3. Make your own food. Then you know what the ingredients are rather than what might come in a package.

## Learn More

*The Whole Soy Story: The Dark Side of America's Favorite Health Food*, by Kaayla Daniel, and thesoydeception.com go in-depth to debunk claims that soy is a health food.

## spoiler alert

*If you think a gluten-free cookie is*
*the healthy choice,*

consider

*that it is still a cookie.*

While gluten-free products may be marginally healthier (depending on your definition of healthy) than their nongluten-free counterparts, consider that they are not necessarily good for you. For example, a gluten-free brownie may still contain sugar and margarine. And just because some brands of potato chips, French fries, beer, and Coke products are labeled gluten-free, doesn't mean they are healthy options. These products are still not the best food choices even without the gluten. Often gluten-free foods are taste-enhanced with extra sweeteners or fats.

Making highly processed foods gluten-free doesn't morph them into the ideal food. They still contain ingredients that are bad for you. Just because Domino's pizza crust is gluten-free doesn't mean that all the other chemicals in the pizza are magically gone and suddenly it is the next wonder antioxidant. Nope, even though gluten-free pizza sounds like it should be good for you, it is still a pizza, and therefore, probably not the best health choice.

> "*Being a 'gluten-free' product does not automatically mean that it is healthy or good for you. Often it is not. For example, Coca-Cola is also gluten-free (and fat free too). However, I do not recommend it.*"
>
> – Dr. Rodney Ford, MD

## Fresh Ideas to Extend Your Expiration Date

Get rid of most grains altogether. Skip the packaged gluten-free foods. Substitute raw zucchini pasta and spaghetti squash for gluten-free noodles. Try out recipes from Paleo, Primal, or raw foodists. These diets don't require ingredients that contain gluten and focus on more natural sweeteners, like honey, maple syrup, and dates.

## Learn More

These websites contain simple recipes that focus on whole, fresh foods without a lot of processing and without gluten because they avoid grains altogether: paleoplan.com/recipes and rawtarian.com.

# spoiler alert

*If you think vegetarianism is*
*a way to get healthy,*

consider

***that this diet is unsustainable without modern supplements, and many vegetarians return to meat eating due to declining health.***

According to Psychology Today, roughly 75 percent of vegetarians eventually return to eating meat. Thirty-five percent of them cite declining health as the deciding factor.[7] There are countless books extolling the virtues of a vegetarian lifestyle, such as *The China Study*, along with vegetarian, vegan, and raw food books. There are also many books extolling the virtues of enormous meat consumption, as in anything related to the Atkins and Paleolithic diets. The people in the middle of the two extremes seem to be the healthiest.

In *Blue Zones: Lessons for Living Longer from the People Who Have Lived the Longest*, a book about different regions with higher-than-normal numbers of centenarians, Dan Buettner notes while studying Sardinia, "Eat a lean plant-based diet accented with meat." Research indicates that it is hard to find a premodern civilization that did not eat some meat or animal products.

In America, meat is often consumed in place of veggies. Nothing says "American" like hamburgers and hotdogs. Meat doesn't need to be the main course of every meal, but to do without it can set you up for iron deficiency anemia along with potential vitamin $B_{12}$ deficiencies. In a vegetarian diet, $B_{12}$ must be obtained from supplementation or the bacteria from unwashed veggies. Yum!

Don't be extreme. Meat doesn't have to be eaten at every single meal. If you are eating it, make sure it is high-quality organic meat. Thomas Jefferson may have had it right when he ate meat as a "condiment to the vegetables."[8]

> "*Eat food. Not too much. Mostly plants.*"
>
> – Michael Pollan, *In Defense of Food: An Eater's Manifesto*

## Fresh Ideas to Extend Your Expiration Date

- Skip the meat substitutes, such as tofu. Most of the time, they are a soy-based protein.
- Use meat as an extra, not as the main course.
- Eat high-quality organic meat and animal products. Nonorganic, conventionally raised animal products are high in hormones, pesticides, and chemicals, and the Omega-3/Omega-6 ratio is often skewed, which leads to inflammation.
- Meat doesn't have to be "certified organic" to be good for you. In fact, pastured animals may be better for you than organic animal products. Animals that are certified organic may be fed diets high in organic corn and soy, which are still unnatural diets for the animals. Pastured animals are often fed diets more congruent to their natural diets, which results in healthier meat. If it is possible, know the people who raises your meat. How they raise and feed them may be more important and healthier than an organic certification.
- Order vegetarian dishes at restaurants unless the meat is specified as organic.
- If you decide vegetarianism is for you, make sure to supplement with iron and $B_{12}$ to avoid deficiencies and health problems.

## Learn More

In *Real Food: What to Eat and Why*, Nina Planck talks about her experiences as a vegetarian and why she went back to meat eating.

*The Omnivore's Dilemma: A Natural History of Four Meals,* by Michael Pollan, is an in-depth look at how food is produced and the health and societal benefits for local, humanely raised, healthily fed animals.

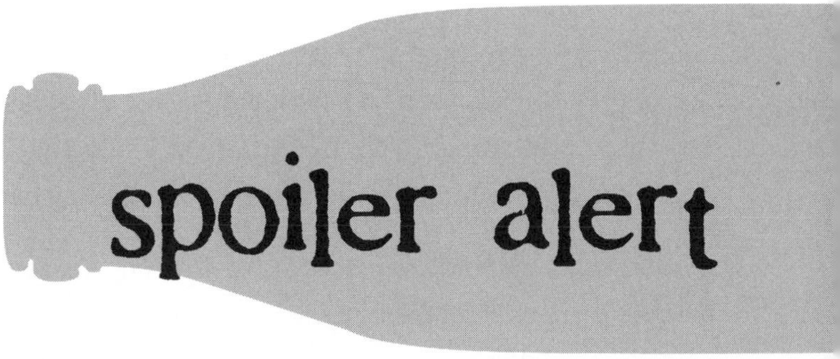

# spoiler alert

*If you think you can only build your bones with the calcium from milk and dairy products,*

consider

*that building strong bones is a multifaceted process.*

Milk advertising is catchy and pervasive, with the "Got Milk?" mustache being one of the top 10 advertising campaigns ever. It's great advertising, but does it tell the whole story? Calcium is a part of building healthy bones, but it's not the whole component, and milk is not the only way to get it.

Studies show that high dairy consumption may not reduce risks to fractures,[9] and the increased intake of dairy products can lead to prostate[10] and ovarian cancer.[11] If dairy is the answer to healthy bones, why doesn't the fracture risk decrease? It may be because more than just calcium goes into building healthy bones. Vitamins A, C, D, $B_{12}$, and K, magnesium, and phosphorous are some of the other important nutrients necessary to build strong bones. Movement and activity are also necessary components.

Veggies can be a good source of calcium: one cup of cooked collard greens contains around 357 mg of calcium, plus the added benefit of other bone-building nutrients, such as vitamin K. Vitamins can have synergistic effects, such as Vitamin D, which helps the body absorb calcium. Without sunlight or extra supplementation, it may be difficult for your body to absorb the calcium you are consuming from dairy products alone. There is controversy that the dietary guidelines for calcium are too high and that ignoring the other nutrients important in bone building may be a detriment. Plus, with the low-fat craze, it is difficult to absorb the fat-soluble vitamins that are present in or fortified into milk, which can contribute to healthy bones.

> *“Those advertisements pushing milk as the answer to strong bones are almost inescapable. But does ‘Got Milk?’ really translate into ‘got strong bones?’”*
>
> – Harvard School of Public Health

## Fresh Ideas to Extend Your Expiration Date

Strong bones are made by a multifactoral approach, not a one-nutrient cure. Even though calcium is the only nutrient emphasized in the “My Plate” government recommendations, it is clearly not the only player in bone development. Don’t just focus on milk and dairy for building strong bones. Focus on staying active with resistance training and getting sunshine. Vary your diet to include many varieties of green leafy veggies: collard greens, mustard greens, kale, and chard, just to name a few. Avoid soy for your calcium intake, even though substituting soy for dairy is a popular trend. Decrease stress levels because increased cortisol decreases calcium absorption. Ignore the catchy dairy advertising “3-A-Day for Stronger Bones” and realize that healthy bones are made from a wide variety of nutrient complexes combined with healthy movement patterns.

Dairy products can be quite controversial these days. Some people are lactose intolerant and cannot digest lactose, and for those concerned about blood sugar levels, milk can cause insulin spikes. Often when choosing dairy, people reach for the low-fat versions. Remember that low-fat/no-fat dairy has added sugars and chemicals to make it taste good and to improve the consistency. Plus, full-fat dairy products allow you to absorb the fat-soluble vitamins contained within.

These are the best ways to consume dairy:

- Raw and fermented full-fat cheese, kefir, and yogurt: Lactose is already partially digested, plus it has the added benefits of increased probiotics (beneficial bacteria to keep our digestive tract healthy).
- Raw, full-fat milk: Pasteurization rids the milk of valuable enzymes and decreases probiotics.
- Choose organic and fermented full-fat products.
- Never consume conventionally produced, inorganic dairy. Why? The cow's diet requires them to be given more antibiotics and growth hormones, such as rBGH, which help the cows produce more milk. Although used in the United States, this growth hormone has been banned in Europe, Canada, Australia, Japan, and other countries because of the potential increased cancer risk in humans and the decreased health of the cows when rBGH is used.

## Learn More

*The Primal Blueprint: Reprogram Your Genes for Effortless Weight Loss, Vibrant Health, and Boundless Energy,* by Mark Sisson, gives compelling lifestyle advice and a balanced approach to dairy. His wildly popular blog at marksdailyapple.com has advice for primal living in a modern world.

# Movement

Movement is free. It requires no cost and very little space. But asking people to move more and get some activity into their daily life is like asking someone to spend money for something they already have, or like trying to give a non-cat lover a cat. Have you ever tried to give away a free cat? It is very difficult, almost as difficult as asking someone to make exercise a long-term, lifestyle choice. Somehow, there are enough hours in a day to surf the Web or watch TV, but for exercise, well, there just isn't the time.

Then there is the question of how to exercise. What are the best ways? How can you maximize your effort? You don't have to exercise several hours a day to benefit, and several hours a day of running or cycling may not be the best for you. It's actually really simple if you consider what your hunter–gatherer ancestors would have done. They would have moved around, doing a lot of running, lifting, pulling, and moving things. They would have been able to participate in active play versus being glued to monitors and TV screens.

Can you be healthy and skinny without exercise? You can be skinny without exercise, but you won't reap the benefits, such as improved health, enhanced quality of life, and all those feel-good chemicals released when you exercise. Weight control is 80 percent diet and 20 percent exercise. Form (the way you look) always follows function (the way you move). If you don't move it, you lose it or you won't develop it because you don't need to. Being active and adding movement to your life is easier than you think and more rewarding than you will ever know. Just try it and see.

# spoiler alert

*If you think good exercise is 30 minutes a day of the same routine,*

## consider

*why your local gym is full of people who can't seem to lose those extra pounds.*

For some reason, the "consistency is king" motto runs rampant in the gym. People trudge away doing the "same old, same old" at the gym and nothing ever changes. Everyone still looks the same and feels the same. Although they may be burning calories, their bodies still lack definition. Why is this?

Bodies are not designed to do the same activity every day. They quickly adapt to this and learn how to use less energy to do the same 30–60 minutes of chugging away at the treadmill, elliptical, or stationary bike. Just like the Specific Adaptation to Imposed Demand (SAID) principle states, your body adapts to the stressors placed on it over time, making it more difficult to achieve results with the same old routine. Don't waste your time on the same old, same old. Diversify your workout portfolio. Excessive aerobic exercise increases your desire for carbohydrates to fuel the muscles because they have been depleted of glucose.

It is important to be well rounded physically, which means you can run fast for an emergency, lift heavy stuff if you need to, and participate in hiking, skiing, sports, mowing the lawn, and gardening. Basically, you need to have the fitness level to perform anything you want to do, without your lack of fitness holding you back.

" *The single thing that comes close to a magic bullet, in terms of its strong and universal benefits, is exercise.* "

– Frank Hu, epidemiologist at Harvard School of Public Health

## Fresh Ideas to Extend Your Expiration Date

Exercise doesn't have to be a drag. Studies have shown exercise can enhance your quality of life. It is not only something that can benefit you in the long term, the mental and physical health benefits can start today. In order to be functionally diverse, you need to include a cardio portion in your physical exercise with interval or sprint training and strength training. Yoga can be a great addition to your weekly routine as it is beneficial for both the body and the mind.

Weekly Activity Plan:

1. Two days of strength training. It doesn't have to take long: 20–30 minutes max. Don't stop for rests. Incorporate full body movements of pushing, pulling, and lifting: squats, lunges, push-ups, pull-ups, tricep dips, and overhead lifts. Don't perform machine bicep curls or machine tricep extensions, which only work one isolated muscle. Do a few sets of body movements at a quick pace until you're fatigued but not injured. Engage your whole body, and you will get more benefit out of your exercise. Every life activity outside of the gym uses a myriad of muscles, so why work one at a time? You will get more benefit for your time and your fitness level if you work them all at once.

2. Three days of intervals. Go as fast as you can for one minute, rest for two minutes and repeat four to eight times. Your total exercise time will be 12–24 minutes. Exercises to choose from include biking (indoor and

outdoor), running, elliptical, swimming, stair running, jumping rope, climbing the StairMaster, and sprinting up hills. Find what works best for you. Some say to sprint for 30 seconds and then rest for four minutes and repeat five times. There isn't a magical number. Do what feels right for your body. How many repetitions and the actual intensity will vary based on your physical fitness level. According to the American College of Sports Medicine, more calories are burned in short, high-intensity exercise. Plus, it can improve your overall athletic performance.

3. One day of long and slow exercise. Hike, run, ride a bike, or practice yoga (great for your mood).

4. One day of rest.

5. Increase your overall activity every day. Walk or bike instead of driving. Get up and move every 15 minutes when you are working. Make your social life revolve around these activities.

## Learn More

At primalhealthyfit.com, there are body weight exercises you can do anywhere, including pictures and modifications. Check out the page on "Basic Movements and Workout Routines."

Marksdailyapple.com presents concise workouts and a great rationale for a more primal diverse workout versus "chronic cardio" workouts.

# spoiler alert

*If you think marathon runners or long distance exercisers are the healthiest individuals,*

consider

*that their bodies may tell a different story.*

"There are few stresses to which the body is exposed that even nearly approach the extreme stresses of heavy exercise." *Guyton Physiology* goes on to say that the metabolism of a person with an extremely high fever increases to about 100 percent above normal. During a marathon, a person's metabolism may increase to 2000 percent above normal.[1] This indicates that heavy, excessive exercise may be more of a stressor than a helper.

Dr. Kenneth Cooper, the father of aerobics, recanted his first stand on excessive aerobics and recommended a lower level of intensity combined with strength training to minimize antioxidant damage to the body in his book, *The Antioxidant Revolution*. If you are creating these free radicals, you have to make healthy lifestyle decisions to counteract them. There is an upper level limit to exercise and if exceeded, could lead to scarring of the heart. Plus, you're putting a lot of stress on your hips, knees, and ankles, especially when running on pavement.

You can't make up for poor eating habits by running marathons. It is found that exercise, such as training for marathons, can lead to weight gain due to an increased desire for carbohydrates. There is a much easier way to stay healthier. Short bursts of exercise (sprinting) are more congruent with what our ancestors would have done. It puts you in better shape overall and gives you more time to incorporate strength training, which will help you develop functional muscles.

> *When people come to me as a cardiologist and say they want to run a marathon, I say, 'OK, do one and cross it off your bucket list and then let's focus on an exercise pattern that's more ideal to producing long-term health benefits and improving your longevity.'*
>
> – James O'Keefe, cardiologist

## Fresh Ideas to Extend Your Expiration Date

Need more proof that short bursts of activity may be healthier? (well, besides the fact that the first ancient Greek runner, whom the marathon is named after, supposedly died after his run) Just look at pictures of sprinters versus marathon runners. Who looks better? Keep in mind they both look healthier than people who don't exercise.

Overexercising or overtraining can lead to increased free radicals and increased stress on the body. If you run marathons or exercise intensely, you will need to increase your other healthy behaviors as well. You can't eat poorly and justify it with exercising because you will need lots of antioxidants to combat heavy exercise. The best way to get antioxidants is from your diet; fresh fruits, veggies, and herbs contain high levels of antioxidants. Your body is an interrelated system, and you need to find a healthy balance in every area of life. Make your activity goal a balanced one—a goal that positively enhances your quality of life, but not to the point where it begins to be a stressor.

Remember, the goal is to be healthy enough and at a fitness level where you can do the things you want to do. You can get greater health benefits from a varied exercise program than from a one-focus exercise plan. A fitness plan that is more congruent with your genetic requirements and based on common sense includes high levels of low-stress activity (walking instead of driving) interspersed with short bursts of high-intensity exercise (running to get somewhere faster or be able to escape danger). Base your exercise patterns on what other mammals in nature do. Generally, they perform low-level activity to find food and water and high-intensity activity when running from perceived danger. Daily, long, high-intensity workouts may cause more wear and tear on your system than you would like. Switch it up. Stay active in a healthy way, so you are able to do all the things you want to do.

## Learn More

*Antioxidant Revolution,* by Kenneth H. Cooper, MD, is a look at the harm caused by excessive overactivity and the benefits of a balanced exercise plan.

In the last 10 years, workout regimens, such as Crossfit, Tabata, and group boot camps, have increased in popularity. You will likely be able to find some in your area.

# spoiler alert

*If you think yoga is only about stretching,*

consider

*that it can actually make you happier.*

Yoga means different things to different people. Some people avoid it due to its religious, philosophical roots, and some people flock to it for its fitness and flexibility benefits. For those concerned about its roots, worry no more. The form of yoga practiced in the United States today is mainly hatha yoga, which is "the variety that centers on postures, breathing, and drills meant to strengthen the body and the mind, as opposed to the yoga of ethics and religious philosophy" (William J. Broad, *The Science of Yoga*).

Physically, yoga can help improve balance, promote less spinal degeneration, decrease inflammation, and help prevent osteoporosis. Unlike most forms of exercise, however, yoga turns you inward rather than outward. Due to the physiological slowing of yoga, it can reduce stress, decrease blood pressure, lower heart rate, boost immunity, and help prevent disease. Numerous studies have been done showing the effects of yoga on the mind with benefits, such as decreased depression, anxiety, tension, and insomnia. Yoga, as it is practiced today, has a little bit of something for everyone. You may try out yoga for the external, physical benefits and find that your mental health is benefiting too.

> “*Yoga has a sly, clever way of short circuiting the mental patterns that cause anxiety.*”
>
> – Baxter Bell, MD

## Fresh Ideas to Extend Your Expiration Date

So how do you get in on this action? It's really simple. Find a yoga studio in your area with a price and schedule that work for you. This way, you get feedback and guidance with the practice in order to do it safely.

Other ways that may fit into your lifestyle but without the feedback is choosing a yoga DVD for beginners, such as Rodney Yee's *A.M. & P.M. Yoga for Beginners* or go online to yogajournal.com for tips and recommendations. Learn to focus on your breath and develop a sense of your body position. How it feels is important, too, and can aid you in preventing injuries and from feeling overwhelmed.

## Learn More

Yogaglo.com gives you access to over 1,000 yoga classes, searchable by skill level or body area you wish to target. Class lengths range from 5 to 90 minutes to fit all schedules. Although it may be clearer to have one-on-one instruction in a class setting, this can be a fabulous resource for at-home learning. It requires a subscription fee, but you can try it for free for 15 days.

If you are looking for yoga in a group setting, then search yogaalliance.org to find registered yoga teachers in your area.

*Yoga for Dummies*, by George Feuerstein, is a helpful introductory book into yoga. With helpful pictures, it introduces yoga to a broad range of age groups.

# spoiler alert

*If you think people who can get by without exercising and manage to stay skinny are healthy,*

## consider

*the "skinny fat."*

"Aww…there's the stick figure. She can eat whatever she wants and never gain a pound."

Picture the people you know who look thin, can eat whatever they want, and never leave the couch. According to research data, people who maintain their weight through diet rather than exercise are likely to have major deposits of internal fat, even if they are otherwise slim.[2] Body scans show that these people (the nonexercisers or super skinny people) have a large deposition of fat around their internal organs and are at risk for insulin resistance and type 2 diabetes. The moral of the story is that you need to exercise, even if you can't tell on the outside.

You can't cheat the system. Exercise builds lean muscle mass, makes for a healthy heart and healthy lungs, and builds bone. Exercise also increases skeletal muscle insulin sensitivity, which causes less demand on your pancreas (giving it a break) for insulin. It is also the best treatment to decrease cortisol, which causes visceral fat deposition (fat around the organs).

In her book *The First 20 Minutes: Surprising Science Reveals How We Can: Exercise Better, Train Smarter, Live Longer*, Gretchen Reynolds interviews Charles Hillman, PhD, from the University of Illinois Neurocognitive Kinesiology Laboratory. He states, "There is no medicine or other intervention that appears to be nearly as effective as exercise" in maintaining or even bumping up a person's cognitive capabilities.[3] Most importantly, exercise is shown to improve your quality of life. Isn't that what it is really all about?

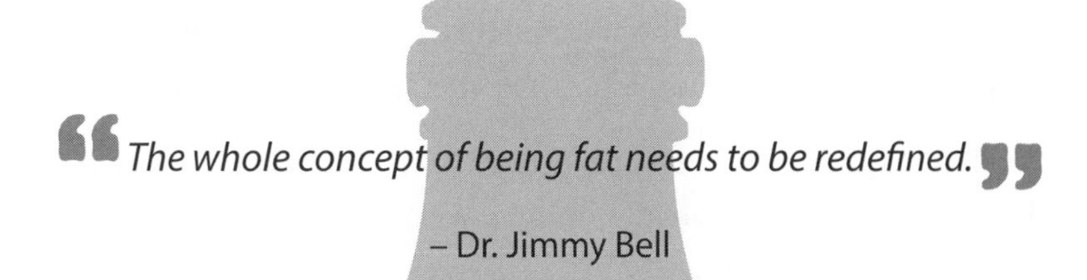

*"The whole concept of being fat needs to be redefined."*

– Dr. Jimmy Bell

## Fresh Ideas to Extend Your Expiration Date

You can be thin or skinny and not be healthy. You can stay thin and look good on the outside without exercising, but that doesn't mean you are healthy. The health risks for the "skinny fat" are similar to those experienced by people who are holding on to a few extra pounds.

For most people, time is the main factor for not making physical activity a part of their lifestyle. In an informative and well-illustrated video espousing the health benefits of exercise, Dr. Mike Evans poses this question, **"Can you limit your sitting and sleeping to just 23 ½ hours a day (or less)?"** This is a good question. We all have 24 hours in a day. Can you only be inactive for 23 ½ hours a day? It only takes 30 minutes of activity a day to see measurable health benefits. Can you spare some time from your inactivity to be active? It just may improve your quality of life.

Looking for ways to add more activity into your life?

- Lead an exercise class. Not only will this make you committed to participating in an activity, but you can also make some extra money.
- Instead of just sitting with your friends and family, try organizing time together around an activity. Go on a walk and then eat or go to an exercise class as a family.
- While talking on the phone, walk around instead of sitting still.
- If you find yourself sitting for long periods of time, get up once an hour and either walk around, do push-ups, tricep dips, squats, or lunges—whatever can be easily done or is appropriate for the environment that you are in. Exercise doesn't have to be done in one big chunk of time. It can be inserted into your day in mini-intervals.

## Learn More

Fun, informative videos on health-related topics are found at myfavouritemedicine.com. A popular one is *23 and ½ Hours*, which shows the benefits of exercise in an entertaining way.

Dr. Mark Hyman talks about "skinny fat" and its health implications on his blog at drhyman.com.

*Drop Dead Healthy: One Man's Humble Quest for Bodily Perfection,* by A. J. Jacobs, provides a very entertaining and funny look at health by a nonhealth care provider, a former "skinny fat" person who made a year-long goal to get healthy. He samples a wide variety of healthy diets and exercise routines.

## spoiler alert

*If you think you can burn off unhealthy extra calories by exercising,*

consider

*that it's a lot harder to accomplish and doesn't quite work that way.*

Consuming unhealthy, extra calories is often justified with "I worked out today; I deserve it," thus creating a psychological reward for exercising. Exercise is also conducted in a way that causes carb cravings, such as daily, long-mileage activity. This type of workout burns up glucose stores, causing these increased carbohydrate cravings. It is common to overestimate calories burned and to underestimate calories consumed. For example, you may burn 300–400 calories on the elliptical machine in 30 minutes, but a 16 oz. Pumpkin Spice Latte (380 calories) at Starbucks will undo it quickly—unless you are a super exerciser, such as Olympian Michael Phelps, with six hours of exercise every day.

Every calorie you eat, whether it be fat, carbohydrate, or protein, is absorbed differently based on its chemical makeup, so you can't just burn off the bad ones. The type of calories you eat makes a difference. The less broken down a food is, the more digestive work your body will do, and thus the more calories will be burned. For example, a complex carbohydrate (such as quinoa) is less broken down before entering the body than white flour is.

The whole muscle-burns-more-than-fat idea is true but only by a little. Fat will burn two calories a day at rest, and muscle will burn six, according to Claude Bouchard of the Pennington Biomedical Research Center. The heavier you are, the higher your basal metabolic rate (how many calories you burn at rest) is. So if you're gaining muscle and losing weight overall, this may equal a few extra potato chips. Not enough to eat that extra pint of Ben and Jerry's.

> “*In general, for weight loss, exercise is pretty useless.*”
>
> – Eric Ravussin, chair in diabetes and metabolism at Louisiana State University and prominent exercise researcher

## Fresh Ideas to Extend Your Expiration Date

- Find a different motivation for exercise than lattes, pizza, or pasta. Instead of visualizing your next meal, visualize how you will feel after you are done and how this will improve your quality of life now and in the future.
- Don't fall into the trap of justifying poor eating decisions with exercise. If you are going to eat something that is bad for you, just do it, but don't justify it. You're lying to yourself, and rationalization can lead to many more unhealthy choices. Make the decision to make poor eating choices consciously, without fooling yourself that they aren't that bad. Once you recognize a bad habit, you can change it. If you keep rationalizing it, you can never make a change.
- Know that exercise is a lifestyle habit that you get to do for the rest of your life. It is as crucial as eating, sleeping, and drinking water. The need for an active lifestyle never goes away.
- Exercise with a goal in mind of feeling good and getting healthier versus how it will make you look.
- The type of exercise that you do, such as running or biking long distances, impacts the food choices you are likely to make. Constant cardio exercise causes an increased craving for carbohydrates. Satisfying these cravings will really cause you to keep on the weight.

## Learn More

In his book, *The Cure for Everything: Untangling Twisted Messages about Health, Fitness, and Happiness*, Timothy Caulfield goes in-depth about exercise and nutrition myths, using himself as a test subject.

The website jonnybowdenblog.com is an interesting commentary from a "rogue nutritionist" and author of nine books. Jonny Bowden's blog, *Exercise Isn't Good for Weight Loss,* is full of good information that is not mainstream yet.

# Emotions

Researchers have long been studying the mind–body connection—the connection that thoughts, emotions, and feelings impact health. Chronic negative stress has been linked to heart disease, hypertension, mental disorders, decreased immune function, and susceptibility to the common cold. Studies show that a healthy mental attitude and strategies to deal with life in an emotionally healthy way impact your resistance to these diseases or can change the disease outcome.

Emotions are experienced on a moment-to-moment basis. Learning how to effectively acknowledge emotions and express them constructively is a key to an internally peaceful life. If you can gain insight into your emotions and thought patterns, you can begin to make healthier decisions and deal with events in your life with more ease.

## spoiler alert

***If you think stress is negative,***

consider

***that it is largely based on perception.***

Stress seems to be everywhere. You are told to avoid it at all times. It is what is making you sick and tired and aging you before your time. What is stress? Hans Seyle, the researcher who coined the word, defined it as the nonspecific response of the body to any demand. This means that stress in your life is not positive or negative, but it is how the body responds to it that makes it positive or negative. It is largely this perception that alters how the body reacts.

When the body feels stress, it initiates the stress hormone cascade, which causes increased heart rate, increased breathing, decreased immune function, increased inflammatory response, increased stress hormones, and weight gain. The stress cascade is very useful in the event of a threat to your survival. The problem is that this stress cascade can be initiated from non-survival-threatening stressors, such as a work deadline or running late to an appointment.

People are often on a high-level of alert with the stress cascade activated constantly. A high state of stress leaves your body's defenses weakened against colds and bacteria and increases the probability of getting sick and developing autoimmune disorders.

How you perceive a situation can affect the stress response in your body. "Life is largely a process of adaptation to the circumstances in which we exist" (Hans Seyle). Most of what is termed stress is what you decide to get anxious and worried about.

> “*People are disturbed not by a thing,*
> *but by their perception of a thing.*”
>
> – Epictetus

## Fresh Ideas to Extend Your Expiration Date

How we perceive stressors is critical and key to how many sick days we have, our recovery time, and our overall quality of life. Stressors, good and bad, are inevitable. Your health is largely determined by how quickly your body is able to respond to the stressor, recalibrate, and return to a state of ease or homeostasis. The best way to handle life issues that present themselves as stressors is to ask, "what is the best way to deal with a negative stressor?" First, decide if it is life threatening.

- If it is life threatening, let your fight-or-flight survival instincts kick in. Run away from a vicious dog or harm-inducing situation.
- If it is not life threatening (includes most situations), then reframe it. Reframing it means to replace a negative thought with a positive one. For example, a consistent stressor may be running late to an appointment. Instead of stressing about it, let the person know you are running late and relax by taking deep breaths, listening to some good music, or just focusing on the moment.

Oftentimes, getting upset and activating the stress cascade are not productive to the situation. Developing better life strategies to maximize eustress and minimize distress will prove more beneficial than chronically activating the internal stress response. As author Michael Hyatt says when faced with a situation that appears bad, "Ask yourself, 'What does this experience make possible?'" Look at it as potential rather than as a problem. Save your stress hormones for survival-threatening occurrences, and improve your quality of life!

## Learn More

*Why Zebras Don't Get Ulcers: The Acclaimed Guide to Stress, Stress-Related Diseases, and Coping*, by Robert M. Sapolsky, is smart, witty, interesting, and science based. Sapolsky takes a physiologic look at how stress affects you and offers strategies for stress reduction.

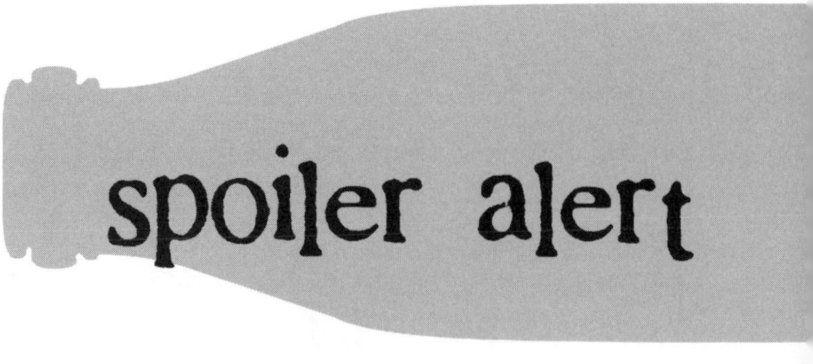

# spoiler alert

*If you think emotions are too difficult to express,*

consider

*how this may affect your health.*

Science doesn't completely understand the mind–body connection: chest pain when feelings are hurt, an ache in the pit of your stomach, gut-wrenching news that makes you nauseated, an endorphin rush when you are happy, butterflies in your stomach, or intense joy that makes it feel like your heart is opening. These are normal and natural emotional responses. In fact, emotional pain involves the same brain regions as physical pain, suggesting the two are inextricably connected.[1]

The problem begins when the emotions get "stuck" through repression, incomplete expression, or continually replay. Emotions seem mysterious because they are invisible, intangible, and you may be unsure of what is the healthy way to approach them. Besides causing you emotional distress and affecting the way you interact with the world, they can sometimes cause bodily pain and symptoms.

Many people have unexpressed emotions or emotional patterns that are not healthy. Oftentimes, they are stymied and can't seem to break through them. It is important to experience emotions fully.

> "*If you don't manage your emotions, then your emotions will manage you.*"
>
> – Doc Childre and Deborah Rozman, PhD

## Fresh Ideas to Extend Your Expiration Date

What does a healthy emotional expression look like?

- Acknowledge, accept, and identify how you are feeling. Acknowledgment requires paying attention and emotional awareness. Don't judge the emotion as good or bad, right or wrong, or whether you should or shouldn't be experiencing it. See if you can identify why you feel the emotion and if there is another underlying emotion. Rather than saying that you are angry, really identify why you are angry. Much of the time, anger is masking as disappointment, hurt, or grief.
- Experience the emotion (happy, sad, mad, grief) without getting caught in the story of why you feel the way you do.
- Breathe. You will notice with intense emotional experiences that you may forget to breathe or your breath will be choppy. Notice where you feel the emotion in your body.
- Express the emotion constructively to yourself first and others if it is necessary.
- Let it go. Once you have processed the emotion, move on. Don't stay stuck on the story behind the emotion.

Pursue lifestyle strategies to process emotions more effectively. Practice relaxation techniques, deep breathing, emotional freedom technique (EFT), journaling, anonymous blogging, meditation, or prayer. Additional outside help may include counseling, neuroemotional technique (NET), or bioenergetic synchronization technique (BEST). Studies suggest that simply exercising equips the brain to better handle emotions. Sometimes emotions can be stuck in muscles. In some forms of movement and body work (such as yoga, massage, chiropractic, acupuncture, tai chi, or qigong), you may experience an emotional release, helping your body heal and reducing pain.

## Learn More

*The Relaxation & Stress Reduction Workbook*, by Martha Davis, Elizabeth Robbins Eshelman, and Matthew McKay, is a comprehensive resource of well-organized, easy-to-practice techniques.

*The EFT Manual,* by Gary Craig, is a user friendly, complete guide for the EFT beginner. Or you can check out eftuniverse.com for a free EFT Mini-Manual.

## spoiler alert

*If you think you cannot control the way you feel,*

consider

*that you may feel that way out of habit.*

Remember what it was like to learn how to ride a bike? First a tricycle, then training wheels, then the magical day when you could freely ride on two wheels. It was a process. This is the same way paths in the brain are formed—with practice. Now as an adult, you still remember how to ride a bike even though you may not have ridden in years. Why? Because the neural paths and muscle memories are still in place.

Forming paths in the brain are like treading a path in the woods where a path has never been before. At first you can't see the path, but every day as you walk it, you can see it more clearly, and it becomes more natural to take. Yet you can get stuck in emotional patterns because you take the same path every day. This may cause you to feel "this is the way I am; I can't change." However, this is not true due to neuroplasticity.

Neuroplasticity (also known as cortical remapping) refers to the ability of the human brain to change as a result of one's experience. The brain is "plastic" and "malleable." Even if it doesn't feel like it at first, making consistent decisions to access a new path leads to change. You don't have to go down destructive, unproductive emotional paths forever. Forge a new path…one that takes you to a better place.

> “*Among other things, neuroplasticity means that emotions, such as happiness and compassion, can be cultivated in much the same way that a person can learn through repetition to play golf and basketball or master a musical instrument, and that such practice changes the activity and physical aspects of specific brain areas.*”
>
> – Andrew Weil

## Fresh Ideas to Extend Your Expiration Date

It may seem like you can't change the way you behave. First, lose the mind-set that you cannot change the way you react. This sets you up for failure. Second, you have to set down new patterns. You can't just get rid of the old ones without replacements.

When you are sad, a common response is to act or express anger, even though sadness is the true emotional feeling. It often doesn't work to tell yourself, "I am just not going to be sad or angry." That is the path you have always taken—the same emotional pathway every day for your entire life. You can't just quit your old emotional responses; you have to replace them with a new behavior. The new behavior may be to express the sadness or anger by telling the person you are sad, by crying, or by another healthier outlet. Write down the new behavior and visualize yourself acting out that new behavior.

When the situation arises again, you will be tempted to choose the well-traveled path to get angry. However, when you begin to choose the new, more productive path you have laid down, then you can begin making healthier emotional decisions. It may seem more difficult at first, but if you stick with it, then it will begin to feel more natural.

As we lay the path with consistent action, then that path will be there for us to access. Making consistent decisions to access a new path leads to change, even if it doesn't feel like it at first.

## Learn More

*The Emotional Life of Your Brain*, by Richard J. Davidson and Sharon Begley, is a heavily researched, in-depth look at the role of emotions in the brain, which helps you to understand your emotions with an explanation of brain chemistry.

*Rewire Your Brain: Think Your Way to a Better Life*, by John B. Arden, is an easily readable book, which describes how your brain can change and how you can easily foster healthy changes. It's the why and how of neuroplasticity and what you can do to enhance it.

# spoiler alert

***If you think you don't have enough,***

## consider

***that you probably have the resources to provide your next meal.***

Most Americans have a lot to be grateful for. Being grateful is one of the best things you can do for your health. It promotes better health, decreases anxiety and depression, improves sleep, gives you higher, long-term satisfaction, and makes you a nicer person to be around.

However, it is a cultural trend to believe you don't have enough things and need more. You may not have everything you want, but you most likely have everything you need. Most Americans have adequate shelter, transportation, clothes, access to clean water, education, and food. You most likely have every tangible object required to survive another day. A lot of people call themselves poor, all the while spending $4 a day at Starbucks. You have a lot to be grateful for. As a cultural rule, Americans have more than most, less than some, but overall, everything they need.

Eighty-four percent of Americans have higher family incomes than their parents had at the same age. Across all levels of the income distribution, this generation is doing better than the one that came before it.[2] That is, the typical person in the bottom 5 percent of the American income distribution is still richer than 68 percent of the world's inhabitants.[3] These statistics should remind you that you have a great life, full of amazing things that you can be grateful for.

> *"The miracle of gratitude is that it shifts your perception to such an extent that it changes the world you see."*
>
> – Dr. Robert Holden

## Fresh Ideas to Extend Your Expiration Date

Make a list of all the things you need. Your needs generally include air, water, food, housing, clothing, and some form of transportation. Do you have access to these things? Awesome. Then you already have a lot to be grateful for, and everything else you have is just extra!

Keep a daily gratitude journal, listing five things you are thankful for. As you are falling asleep at night, count your blessings instead of sheep. Make it a point to tell your partner or family something you appreciate about them every day. Make gratitude a part of your life and notice how it changes you for the better.

Remind yourself daily of the things you have rather than the things you do not have.

## Learn More

*Thanks! How Practicing Gratitude Can Make You Happier*, by Robert A. Emmons, is a well-researched, well-written book on the subject of gratitude and how it can impact your life for the better. It includes relevant tips on how to apply gratitude. This book is one of several titles the author has written on the subject.

At happyrambles.com, you can keep an online gratitude journal free of charge. Every day you will get an e-mail with the question "What are you grateful for today?" You can reply and the entry will be stored forever, for your eyes only. It's a great way to make gratitude a part of your daily ritual.

# Chemical Peer Pressure

The myths in this section are about chemicals commonly used in everyday life. Most people agree with the saying "better living through chemistry." Sometimes science improves the quality of life, such as in the case of sanitation or emergency care. Sometimes it doesn't, as in the case of the atom bomb and nuclear disasters. Not every new chemical compound made in a laboratory is healthy for people or the environment. Since World War II, at least 80,000 compounds have been invented and dispersed into the environment, with only a portion tested for human toxicity.[1]

To an extent, you decide how many chemicals you allow in your daily life. It starts with you and the products you choose to purchase and bring into your home. As an individual, you have a choice about the chemicals you allow on your skin, in your home, in the water you drink, and ultimately in your body. This section reveals common chemicals in your environment, some of which you may not even know are present.

## spoiler alert

*If you think what you put on your skin isn't important,*

consider

*that your skin absorbs what you put on it.*

Your skin is actually your body's largest organ. Oftentimes, it is viewed only as a separation or protection from the outside world. However, it also absorbs from the outside world, which is why pain patches, birth control patches, and nicotine patches work. Don't put anything on your skin that you wouldn't want to be inside of your body.

Studies show that different substances absorb at different rates, with certain places on the body being more absorbable. You can estimate about a 60 percent absorption rate overall with increased absorbability on the face, underarms, abdomen, behind the ears, and 100 percent absorbability on the genitals.[2] Be careful! The ingredients in the products you put on your body will likely end up inside of your body.

Parabens, phthalates, and petrolateum are all common ingredients in body care, soaps, lotions, and cosmetics. Parabens and petrolateum have been linked to breast cancer, and phthalates have been linked to disrupting the endocrine system, yet they are still allowed in personal care products. These are just a few of the many chemicals in your personal care products.

Reducing the toxic load in the products you use on your hair and skin is a choice that you can make. You cannot always control the environmental toxins around you, but what you put on your skin is something that you can control.

> *I got rid of half my [beauty products]. When you look at the ingredients and you can't pronounce them? That's a really strong indication that you don't want to put it on your lips.*
>
> – Julia Roberts on *Oprah*

## Fresh Ideas to Extend Your Expiration Date

Whatever you put on your skin is being absorbed into your body. It is your decision which products you use. It is your toxic load. Some chemicals found in our environment are there because of the choices of others. You can choose the chemicals that go in your skin care products.

Get rid of and don't buy synthetic fragrances or chemicals that you can't pronounce. A good rule is to not put on your skin what you would not put in your mouth. Or if you can't pronounce it, then it may not be good for you. There may be some exceptions, but as a general rule, it is good advice. Say no to most popular brands of makeup, shampoo, soap, deodorant, and lotion. They often have ingredients you wouldn't want to end up in your body.

Help yourself reduce your toxic load:

- Go outside the mainstream grocery store for your body care. Choose organic but really read the labels because they can be very tricky. Things that look healthy upon closer label inspection are oftentimes not very healthy. For example, body products that are labeled "Natural" often contain toxic chemicals but are marketed to look healthy.
- Make your own stuff using a good base and quality essential oils.
- Use simple things, such as coconut oil, for a body moisturizer. Do some research. It is really amazing how easy it is to use natural, everyday products for body care.

## Learn More

*What's in This Stuff? The Hidden Toxins in Everyday Products and What You Can Do about Them*, by Patricia Thomas, is a comprehensive resource for what's in common products from toiletries and cosmetics to household products and pet supplies. It includes alternatives to common products, plus an A–Z glossary of common chemicals.

Do-it-yourself books, such as *Natural Beauty at Home: More Than 250 Easy-to-use Recipes for Body, Bath, and Hair*, by Janice Cox, have recipes for making your own, organic, good-for-you products. An easy Internet search of do-it-yourself information on whatever product you are looking for (such as natural shampoo) will lead you to a plethora of recipes with reviews.

# spoiler alert

*If you think applying sunscreen is always the healthiest choice,*

consider

*that you need vitamin D from the sun.*

Sun used to be in. Now it's out. Real tan used to be in. Now it has been replaced by spray tans. Sunscreen is in—almost to the point that everyone is scared to be without it. The fear comes, not from being burned, but from the possibility of developing skin cancer.

What does the sun do? Fundamentally, it provides all life on earth. It is the earth's primary source of energy. It helps grow food, provides antiseptic properties, and along with the moon, controls the tides. Basically, it's essential to all life.

The sun causes our bodies to produce vitamin D. This is not just any vitamin; it is also a hormone and is extremely important to bone health. It helps the body absorb calcium, control inflammation, and activate the immune system. Plus, it can assist in the prevention of numerous forms of cancer, especially breast,[3] colorectal,[4] ovary, and kidney. It is extremely important, but people can't get it if they are covered in sunscreen every second. The ingredients from sunscreen, such as oxybenzone, nano-scale zinc oxide, avobenzone, and benzophenone, to name a few, are toxic and may contribute to cancer as well.

You can get small amounts of vitamin D from foods, such as fish and egg yolks, but it is almost impossible to get all of it from diet alone. You need the sun, so don't be scared of it. Go get your vitamin D, but just do so responsibly.

> "*Light is the basic component from which all life originates, evolves, and is energized. Light and health are inseparable.*"
>
> – Ken Ceder, former codirector of Hippocrates Health Institute

## Fresh Ideas to Extend Your Expiration Date

What does responsible sun exposure look like? Well, it does not involve baking in the sun for hours on end. What it does involve is direct sunlight 10–15 minutes a day with no sunscreen for fair skinned individuals and up to 60 minutes a day for darker skinned individuals. It does not involve tanning beds either. Since July 2010, tanning beds have been taxed an extra 10 percent due to their ability to cause an increase in melanoma.

You need to supplement with vitamin $D_3$ (the active form) on days you are not exposed to the sun. The recommended daily allowance for vitamin D is 600 IU. However, this is a recommendation that keeps you from getting rickets, not for helping you thrive. Remember, vitamin D is a fat-soluble vitamin, so for better absorption, supplement it with a meal where fat is ingested. A sublingual (taken under the tongue) vitamin D is the best one to take because it immediately enters systemic circulation, versus an oral ingested vitamin D, which is absorbed in the digestive tract.

If you are going to be out in the sun for a long time and need some protection, invest in natural or "green" sunscreens. They protect you from the sun without adding toxins to your skin.

## Learn More

A quality, sublingual source of vitamin D is located at innatechoice.com.

A quick read about the power of vitamin D to treat conditions and why it is so necessary is *Power of Vitamin D: A Vitamin D Book That Contains the Most Comprehensive and Useful Information on Vitamin D Deficiency, Vitamin D Level*, by Sarfraz Zaidi, MD.

# spoiler alert

*If you think the flu shot makes you healthy,*

consider

*that its active ingredients are the results of an educated guessing game.*

Most people think that the flu shot has been tested and will prevent you from getting the flu. Straight from the label of the 2012–2013 Flulaval vaccine: "…there have been no controlled trials adequately demonstrating a decrease in influenza disease after vaccination with Flulaval."[5] From the Center for Disease Control website: "It is not possible to predict how well the vaccine and circulating strains will be matched in advance of the influenza season, and how this match may affect vaccine effectiveness."[6]

The flu vaccine is basically a guess, an amalgamation of the three viruses that research indicates are most likely to be present in the next flu season and is prepared well before the flu season. The University of Minnesota conducted a study in which they researched all the flu vaccine studies from 1967–2011. They concluded "that most flu vaccines provide only moderate protection against influenza, and in some years barely make a difference at all."[7] The flu vaccine had a 59 percent success rate in preventing the flu.[8] That is a failing score in most institutes of higher education.

Yet, if you look up ways to prevent the flu, it is often number one on the list. The flu shot has good marketing, but that does not necessarily mean it is effective.

> “*I really believe your immune system takes care of a lot of things. Even if you've been exposed to the flu, you don't have to get it.*”
>
> – Erica Brownfield, MD, and professor of internal medicine at Emory University School of Medicine, Atlanta, GA

## Fresh Ideas to Extend Your Expiration Date

What are the best ways to prevent the flu?

- Keep your immune system healthy.
- Wash your hands. This is basic advice but extremely important.
- Get plenty of rest, water, and sunlight (vitamin $D_3$ if you don't have access to sun).
- Consume lots of fresh veggies. Try for two to three servings at every meal.
- Be active every day.
- Decrease your stress load. Learn to say yes only to things that matter.

## Learn More

In general, vaccinations can be a controversial issue with heavily disputed arguments on both sides. It is important to make educated, informed decisions about vaccines. You have to decide what is right for you and your family.

spoiler alert

*If you think fluoride is healthy to consume,*

consider

*that too much of it can cause health problems.*

Ever wonder why your toothpaste label says: "Warning: Keep out of the reach of children under 6 years of age. If more than used for brushing is accidentally swallowed, get medical help or contact a Poison Control Center right away." Fluoride, a naturally occurring element, can be dangerous if consumed in high doses. The risk is high, especially for children, and contributes to dental fluorosis (cosmetic damage to teeth, causing brown or white spots) and skeletal fluorosis (risk of bone fractures). Low-level topical doses are thought to prevent tooth decay, but high-level systemic doses (as in drinking water or from swallowing fluoridated toothpaste) are thought to contribute to health problems.

The 2010 statistics from the Center of Disease Control state that 73.9 percent of the drinking water in the United States is fluoridated either naturally or artificially. In 2011, due to an alarming increase in dental fluorosis in two out of five adolescents, the United States decreased the amount of fluoride in the water. Studies done in Europe, where all countries do not participate in water fluoridation, show a decline in dental decay regardless if the country fluoridates its water.[9]

Studies done in areas with high levels of fluoride in the water have shown decreased IQ levels in children. It is shown to have effects on the brain, nervous system, thyroid, and it may contribute to certain types of cancer. With the addition of fluoride to water come small amounts of arsenic, lead, and radionuclides.[10] The EPA says fluoride is a chemical with "substantial evidence of developmental neurotoxicity."[11]

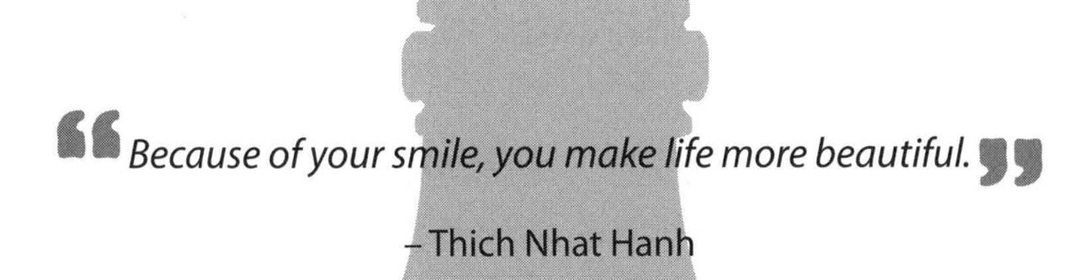

> *Because of your smile, you make life more beautiful.*
>
> – Thich Nhat Hanh

## Fresh Ideas to Extend Your Expiration Date

Without clear proof that adding fluoride to the water supply is safe and because of the inability to monitor how much is consumed, fluoridation should be an option, not the rule. The source of the fluoride added to drinking water may be a concern. It is an industrial waste from the production of phosphate fertilizer. Putting it in the water eliminates the need for toxic waste disposal.

Fluoride doesn't appear to protect teeth through ingestion. It is believed to only work topically. If you feel fluoride is necessary and protective, then you can choose to get it from toothpastes, gels, and mouthwashes. To avoid water fluoridation, filter your tap water with a good quality filter that removes fluoride.

How are cavities and tooth decay produced? Cavities are produced when the plaque on teeth interacts with sugars and starches, causing the enamel to breakdown. Fluoride is not the only step you can take towards tooth health. Other proven steps:

1. Limit sugars, including soda, juices, milk, and refined carbohydrates from breads, pastas, and flour. Their interaction is what causes cavities

in the first place. Even diet sodas, which contain no sweeteners, are acidic and may cause decay as well.

2. Stop smoking. Smoking has been linked to poor oral hygiene and cavities, plus it's just not good for your overall health.

**Bonus Health Tip: While on the subject of teeth, SMILE! It makes you feel better. Researchers say that just the act of putting a smile on your face can elevate your mood.**

## Learn More

*The Fluoride Deception*, by Christopher Bryson, is a well-referenced guide to the story of fluoride in America—complete with conspiracies and cover-ups, making the study of fluoride interesting.

# spoiler alert

*If you think guzzling eight glasses of bottled water a day is the healthiest choice,*

consider

*that there may be healthier options for you and the planet.*

Staying hydrated is essential and can enhance your mental clarity, increase your feeling of fullness, and keep the digestive tract moving. Sometimes you get hunger signals simply because you are dehydrated. There is a big debate about the best drinking water: tap water, bottled water, or filtered water.

As of 2010, there were 60,000 chemicals in use in the United States, with many chemicals making it into the drinking water supply. The Safe Drinking Water Act only regulates 91 contaminants in tap water.[12] Studies have shown bottled water is not well regulated, may have more contaminants than filtered water, or is just filtered tap water. In 2011, US bottled water sales totaled 9.1 billion gallons.[13] According to Charles Fishman, author of *The Big Thirst*, "…in the half-liter size Americans find so appealing, that comes to 222 bottles of water for each person in the country."[14] Skip the middleman. Save the plastic waste of the water bottles, and invest in a filtering system for your tap. By filtering it yourself, you can know what isn't in your water.

How much water should you drink? Ideally you should obtain a large amount of water content from your food. Local, fresh-picked veggies and fruits have significantly higher water content than their weary, traveling supermarket friends. If you are not eating high water-content foods, then drinking eight glasses of water, or half your body weight in ounces, is probably a good thing to do. It's not always mandatory if you are getting plenty of water from your diet.

> *Water and air, the two essential fluids in which all life depends, have become global garbage cans.*
>
> – Jacques Cousteau

## Fresh Ideas to Extend Your Expiration Date

The take-home message is to focus on getting part of your water from high water-content fresh fruits and veggies. The rest you can get from filtered tap water. Having a clean water supply will help to reduce your overall toxic load. Reverse osmosis with a superior carbon filter is the best process. Whole house filters are the best due to absorbability of water toxins by the body through the skin. Pure, clean, filtered water is the best beverage choice.

If you are bored with the taste of water, add mint, lime, or lemon for flavor. Herbal teas can be a great addition as well, adding health benefits from the herbs. Just avoid the herbal teas with natural flavors in the ingredients. Often these "natural ingredients" are made from chemicals, not from anything natural.

Helpful tip: Don't wait until meal time to catch up on your water intake. Chinese medicine indicates that large amounts of water will dilute digestive enzymes and secretions, and food nutrients won't be effectively extracted. A small amount of water at a meal may be helpful, but if you stay hydrated all day, you will not need to ingest large amounts of water at meals.

## Learn More

For a resource for what is happening to your water supply, visit projects.nytimes.com/toxic-water to see how it is regulated and access additional links to more water information.

Find information for selecting the best type of water filter for your home and your needs at ewg.org/tap-water/getawaterfilter.

There are some natural springs in the United States where you can collect and bottle your own water. Check out findaspring.com to see if there is one near you.

# Popular Health Beliefs

This section touches on popular health beliefs perpetuated by tradition, media, and well-meaning people. These common ideas that personal health care should be entrusted to someone outside of yourself, such as the government or a doctor, are leading to an increase in health care costs and a decrease in the quality of life. Making your health a priority is up to you.

The general perception of health prevention is that it requires screenings and diagnostic tests. While these measures may prevent disease progression, they do not prevent the disease from occurring, plus they are generally costly. The prevention addressed in this book is the prevention of the disease before it begins by making healthy lifestyle decisions.

# spoiler alert

*If you think it costs a lot to be healthy,*

consider

*that it costs more to be unhealthy.*

Every time you exchange money to purchase entertainment, an activity, food, or beverage, you vote for something that will take you toward health or away from it. Sometimes those votes cost more initially. For example, high-quality food (well-raised animal products and organic, local food) usually costs more than highly processed, mass produced food from a faraway land.

Health care spending is generally focused on treating a disease after it has been diagnosed. The projected 2023 costs for chronic disease are 4.1 trillion dollars.[1] Seven out of 10 US deaths are currently caused from chronic disease,[2] which is predominantly linked to lifestyle choices. The traditional health care system in the United States is focused on treating the complications of disease without forethought to the prevention.

There are signs of hope that prevention may one day be valued. For example, research is beginning to focus on the cost savings of simple health steps. Research in the United Kingdom demonstrates millions of dollars would be saved due to decreased health problems if breast feeding rates were to increase.[3] Millions of dollars could be saved if children were to breast feed, like they did for thousands of years before the invention of formula. Simple, natural, common sense health measures are proving to be healthier and more cost effective than unnatural interventions. Prevention of health problems is more cost effective than treating the disease process after it occurs.

> *“Every time you spend money, you're casting a vote for the kind of world you want.”*
>
> – Anna Lappe

## Fresh Ideas to Extend Your Expiration Date

You can vote with your finances to move towards a healthy life or towards an unhealthy life. It initially costs more to vote for good food, quality water, less-toxic cleaning supplies, more natural skin and body care, a gym membership, or activities that are nourishing to your life, such as photography, art, music, and dance. It initially costs more to take care of yourself with chiropractic, acupuncture, massage, and other forms of bodywork. The payoff is down the road of life where you can visibly see that your vote mattered and counted with your improved quality of life.

It is more cost effective to maintain your vehicle than to let it run out of oil and have to fix or replace a burned-out engine. Prevention is less dramatic than curing. Curing a disease or saving a life against all odds is sensational, generally costly, and makes a good story. Prevention is not as glamorous, but it is exciting to not spend your money, time, or energy looking for a cure. Redirect the money that you are spending on cures, over-the-counter prescriptions, copayments, fast food, alcohol, and cigarettes, and invest it either in long-term money investments (such as an IRA) or back into your health in the form of good-for-you food, beverages, and lifestyle choices.

How you move, how you feel, and your general attitude about life are influenced by the decisions you made yesterday. Likewise, tomorrow's quality of life will be influenced by the investments of today. It will show in the quality of your older years. You pay now or you most likely will pay more later. You can thrive as you age or you can merely survive.

## Learn More

Learn more about the value of prevention and true wellness in the book *The Wellness & Prevention Paradigm* by Dr. James L. Chestnut. It is full of great analogies and research to switch your paradigm of what it is to be truly healthy.

# spoiler alert

*If you think you have to shop in a health food store to eat healthy,*

consider

*healthier, less-structured options.*

Designated "health" food stores can be expensive. It may be hard to get excited about shopping at them (even though I still do) when you spend so much more money to shop there. It is possible to vote economically with your money. A very popular blog, "100 Days of Real Food," shows that it can be done with a family of four.

Some things are easier to buy at health food stores. However, fruits, veggies, local animal products, local honeys, and many more things can be found in less structured, more informal, local options: Community Support Agriculture (CSA) boxes, your own garden, farmers markets (seasonal and year round), produce stands, foraging, and food co-ops. Some options, such as gardening, involve getting up close and personal with your food, while other options allow you to maintain a very safe distance from your food (buying versus picking it yourself). Get out of the health store and try something new and more economical. By getting out of the health food store and going local, you may benefit yourself, reduce environmental waste from long distance travel, and eat a fresher product that tastes better with more nutritional value and water content.

> "*Ultimately, we have the food system that we have, because that's what we want.*"
>
> – Joel Salatin, Polyface Farms

## Fresh Ideas to Extend Your Expiration Date

Opportunities to step out of the health food store abound. Research places around you where you can obtain good quality produce and animal products year round. (Some outside-the-box health food options are seasonal.)

- Buy in bulk during the growing season from local farms or places like azurestandard.com and split with friends. Or preserve it for later with good food preservation techniques, such as drying, freezing, and canning.
- CSA boxes are delivered weekly, providing opportunities for local produce with a variety you may never purchase on your own.

## Learn More

Nationwide websites, such as localharvest.org and foodroutes.org, list farms and farmers markets near you.

*Eat Where You Live: How to Find and Enjoy Fantastic and Local Sustainable Food No Matter Where You Live*, by Lou Bendrick, provides resources for finding food outside the health food store or grocery store no matter where you live.

# spoiler alert

*If you think improving your health is time consuming and difficult,*

consider

*the productivity loss and inconvenience of being sick.*

Making healthy decisions requires the same amount of time as making unhealthy ones. It is only a matter of where you put your focus. Everyone is allotted the same 24 hours. It is the focus of those 24 hours that leads in the direction of either better health or more sickness. The perception that it takes more time to be healthy may just be an excuse for something you don't really want to do.

Time is viewed as one of the most precious commodities next to money. Time is free, abundant, and available to all. The awesome thing about time is that you get to choose how you spend it. You can either spend time creating a healthy life now, while you feel good, or try to create it after you become sick.

If you wait, you may be spending your time on remedies, doctors' visits, and tests. You won't feel like being productive at home or on the job. You won't have the energy to cultivate relationships with your friends and family. You will spend your time trying to regain your health. Why not invest the time in creating health today instead of spending time trying to regain it later?

> “*Those who think they have no time for healthy eating will sooner or later have to find time for illness.*”
>
> – modified from Edward Stanley (1826–1893) from *The Conduct of Life*

## Fresh Ideas to Extend Your Expiration Date

How you spend your time is a great reflection of what you value. If you value health, you will choose to spend time making healthy decisions. If you value a clutter-free, simple home environment, you will spend time creating that. It is all about what you choose to create.

Choose to create a healthy environment—one where there are good strategies for coping with life stressors, good strategies to implement healthy food, and good strategies to encompass healthy movement patterns. The time you invest in making quality health decisions will pay off with an improved quality of life both now and in the future.

Starting today is key. Health is an investment, and with all investments, the sooner you begin, the more it compounds, and the less you have to catch up. As a wise proverb says, "The best time to plant a tree is 20 years ago. The second best time is now."

## Learn More

A couple of books on how to implement healthy changes easily: *Better Each Day: 365 Expert Tips for a Healthier, Happier You,* by Jessica Cassity, includes 365 daily tips to make you healthier.

If you want a weekly style of easily manageable changes, choose *52 Small Changes: One Year to a Happier, Healthier You* by Brett Blumenthal. Both authors present easy, healthy changes that you can continually make.

> *American's fear only one thing...inconvenience.*
>
> – George Naylor in *Fresh: New Thinking about What We're Eating*, a documentary

# spoiler alert

*If you think, "I will sleep when I am dead,"*

consider

*that this mentality may get you there sooner.*

Sleep is often the first thing to be discarded when life gets busy. Kids, life, work, relationships, and exercise get attended to first and sleep is discarded. It should be a nonnegotiable, right up there with good hygiene. However, it is oftentimes discarded like leftover French fries. What is the reason for the ambivalence about sleep? Maybe it is because in the American workaholic culture, it appears that nothing important is happening while sleeping. The truth is your body is repairing and rejuvenating. You are not wasting time by sleeping. In fact, you are likely increasing your productivity by being well-rested and not feeling continually lost in a dense, sleepy fog.

Sleep is when the brain recharges. It is like a reset button for the body. Enough sleep can boost creativity, lift your mood, sharpen attention, improve your performance, and make you a better person to be around by decreasing irritability. It will improve your immune system, make you less susceptible to disease, and decrease risks for heart disease, diabetes, and weight gain. Adequate sleep is pretty much awesome. Plus, it may very realistically increase your personal safety by simply decreasing car accidents. One hundred thousand accidents a year are estimated to be caused by drowsy driving.

> “*Without enough sleep, we all become tall two year olds.*”
>
> – JoJo Jensen, *Dirt Farmer Wisdom*

## Fresh Ideas to Extend Your Expiration Date

Restructure your life to achieve seven to nine hours of sleep a night. This is often the biggest challenge. Sleep is decreased in order to achieve more things; however, sleeping more may actually improve your performance and increase your concentration and efficiency. Say yes only to the important things. Sleep is one of those important things.

Set a time to go to bed and a time to wake up every day. Your body secretes certain hormones to help you go to sleep and hormones to help you wake up. Get your body in a rhythm. A lack of a structured schedule can feel like perpetual jet lag.

Declutter the room you sleep in so it's a restful place where your body can wind down. Dim the lights and have a no-electronics zone one hour before you go to bed: no TVs, laptops, video games, phones, or other lighted devices. Our bodies used to go to sleep with the sun and wake up with it. Create the environment by setting the "sleep mood."

If the inability to fall asleep is one of your challenges, try relaxation techniques, such as progressive relaxation, guided sleep imagery, or deep relaxation at umm.edu/sleep /relax_tech.htm.

## Learn More

Don't go any longer without getting restful, quality sleep. A website for designing optimal sleep environments is found at bedroom.sleepfoundation.org.

*Good Night: The Sleep Doctor's 4-Week Program to Better Sleep and Better Health,* by Michael Breus, PhD, contains sleep information, including a four-week sleep boot camp with a different direction every day.

*No More Sleepless Nights,* by Peter Hauri, PhD, and Shirley Linde, PhD, is a slightly less recent publication but a great book if you have a more difficult time falling asleep.

# spoiler alert

***If you think your doctor, your insurance company, or the government will keep you healthy,***

**consider**

***that no one cares about your well-being like you do.***

"When it comes to your health, you need to become the expert because it is your day-to-day decisions that have the greatest impact on your health and quality of life," according to Dr. James Chestnut, author of *The Wellness Paradigm*. Medical doctors as a general rule cannot "fix" you. They can give you a drug or perform a surgery that keeps you from expressing symptoms, but true healing comes from addressing what created the disease process in the first place.

The doctor is with you for a brief time. A 10-minute office visit is not enough time for the doctor to untangle the lifestyle choices you have or haven't made. A prescription drug can change your symptoms but will do little to address the cause of them. Drugs should not be a substitute for examining the real cause of symptoms, which are oftentimes poor lifestyle choices. The Medicare and Medicaid guidelines (the government's standard of health care) offer no reimbursement for preventative care.

Health insurance could easily be renamed "disease insurance." Most insurance plans only offer sickness care, which is payment for services after you become sick. There is no reimbursement for being proactive and preventing disease with quality lifestyle choices. The responsibility of wellness lies squarely on your shoulders. Making good lifestyle decisions has to be your choice.

> "*When you take charge of your life, there is no longer need to ask permission of other people or society at large. When you ask permission, you give someone veto power over your life.*"
>
> – Albert Geoff

> *"Health insurance has as much to do with being healthy as life insurance has to do with being alive. If you rely on an insurance company's recommended plan for your health care needs, we hope you have good life insurance."*
>
> – Author Unknown

## Fresh Ideas to Extend Your Expiration Date

No one has as much interest in your health care as you do. Healthy and unhealthy decisions add up over time. It is impossible to undo a lifetime of unhealthy decisions in one doctor's visit, one vitamin, one pill, or one chiropractic visit. Sustained action over time leads to results. It is a responsibility that begins and ends with you.

You don't have to be sick or have an unwanted diagnosis to add healthy choices to your life. Some of the best ways to enhance your life are through healthy foods, exercise, healthy emotional patterns, yoga, meditation, chiropractic, massage, and acupuncture. All of the above will optimize your potential and help you tune into your body.

Getting healthy is as simple as adding healthy lifestyle changes. Seriously, that is all it takes. It doesn't have to be overnight, and it doesn't have to be all or none. For example, add a fresh fruit or vegetable before every meal or add 30 seconds of deep breathing into your daily routine. If your work involves increased sitting, set an hourly timer. Then when it goes off, get up, stretch, and walk around. You can add healthy lifestyle changes, and over time they will become second nature to you. Taking care of yourself is a decision that you can make without relying on the government, an insurance company, or a doctor.

## Learn More

*How We Do Harm: A Doctor Breaks Ranks about Being Sick in America,* by Otis Webb Brawley, MD, is an informative look from the director of the American Cancer Society on how medical treatment is decided, to whom it is given, and its effectiveness.

# spoiler alert

***If you think wellness screenings, or "preventative care" as the insurance companies define it, keep you healthy,***

**consider**

***that they are merely diagnostic and do not change your health status.***

Dental X-rays don't prevent tooth decay; they reveal it. Mammograms don't prevent cancer; they reveal lumps. Scans, screenings, exams, and imaging don't prevent disease; they only reveal it after it has begun. These wellness screenings for high blood pressure, cholesterol levels, and blood sugar, don't impact the disease that is creating it. They merely detect it. Insurance covers preventative health screenings, such as mammograms and colonoscopies. They tell you if you have disease, not how to keep you healthy.

The goal of a health screening is not to prevent disease but to detect it before it gets worse. This detection is not prevention. A person isn't always well just because the screening comes back with a clean bill of health. Research shows that some forms of cancer may take 20 years to develop before they are detectable.

You have been informed that if you are screened for a disease, it can be prevented. That is simply untrue. A dental X-ray may reveal a cavity, but it doesn't prevent it from occurring. The progression may be prevented, such as filling a cavity before having the tooth pulled. Screenings aren't necessarily bad, unless they are exposing you to ionizing radiation, which in that case, the costs would outweigh the benefits. Preventative screenings are an oxymoron. Screenings may prevent disease progression; they don't prevent disease.

> “*People in America may not live longer, but we sure do a better job taking pictures (scans) of them dying.*”
>
> – Otis Brawley, MD

## Fresh Ideas to Extend Your Expiration Date

- Get health screenings if you think they are necessary. They will not prevent disease but may keep the disease from progressing further.
- Don't depend on a health screening to tell you if you are healthy or not.
- Be proactive rather than reactive and implement healthy changes now.

## Learn More

*Over Diagnosed: Making People Sick in the Pursuit of Health,* by Dr. H. Gilbert Welch, provides an in-depth look at the risks and pitfalls versus the benefits of disease screenings for healthy individuals. He takes a look at excessive diagnosis, changing diagnostic values, and the ability to do harm with overtreatment.

## spoiler alert

*If you think birth is a medical emergency,*

consider

*that the world has been repopulating for centuries without much interference.*

Without a doubt, there can be high-risk pregnancies and birth emergencies where medical interventions are highly necessary. Although overall, birth is not the medical emergency that the Western culture makes it out to be. The Western view of birth tells a lot about the way the culture views life in general. Birth is a normal physiologic process that all other mammals undertake, mostly without intervention. Instead, this culture treats it as a process to be highly monitored, planned, and micromanaged with drugs, shots, inductions, preplanned births, ultrasounds, screenings, and tests.

The United States spends more on health care than any other country and more on maternal health than any other type of hospital care. However, it is ranked 50 in maternal mortality and 41 in neonatal mortality worldwide.[4] These rankings put us behind such countries as the Czech Republic and Cuba.

Currently, about one-third of all American babies are delivered surgically via C–sections. This number is extremely high with the World Health Organization, which reports that the optimal C–section rate for a country is between 5 and 10 percent. Rising C–section rates are linked to a variety of causes, including the health of the mother and baby, convenience for the doctor and mother, fear of malpractice suits, and other interventions, such as planned inductions and epidurals. The cultural perception of birth needs to change to reflect that birth is a normal physiological process, and intervention with that process does not always equal health for the mother or the baby.

> “*Birth is not an emergency. It is simply an emergence.*”
>
> – Jeannine Parvati Baker

## Fresh Ideas to Extend Your Expiration Date

Evidence in support of the safety of planned home births for healthy, low-risk women continues to grow.[5] Shift your perception about the process of birth. Educate yourself and the people in your life on what natural birth can look like. Before pregnancy, educate yourself with resources about midwives, doulas, birthing centers, and home birth. Know that you have other options that may lie outside the cultural "normal."

## Learn More

The documentary, *The Business of Being Born*, is an insightful look into the medicalization of birth and other birthing options besides the hospital route.

*Active Birth: The New Approach to Giving Birth Naturally*, by Janet Balaskas, and *The Other Baby Book: A Natural Approach to Baby's First Year*, by Megan McGrory Massaro and Miriam J. Katz, give balanced, holistic childbirth advice.

# Chiropractic

Although medical doctors and doctors of chiropractic are separate and distinct, both have high-level educations. The main difference between medical doctors and chiropractors is in what they offer the patients who come to see them. Medical doctors often address sickness and pain with drugs or surgery. Chiropractors offer physical and spinal adjustments and often lifestyle modifications. Most chiropractors do not prescribe medication.

Most people assume that chiropractors have less of an education than medical doctors. Based on the chart on the next page, that is clearly not the case. The class hours for basic science comparisons were compiled and averaged, following a review of curricula of 18 chiropractic colleges and 22 medical schools.

| Chiropractic College | | Medical School |
|---|---|---|
| 456 | Anatomy/Embryology | 215 |
| 243 | Physiology | 174 |
| 296 | Pathology | 507 |
| 161 | Chemistry/Biochemistry | 100 |
| 145 | Microbiology | 145 |
| 408 | Diagnosis | 113 |
| 149 | Neurology | 171 |
| 56 | Psychology/Psychiatry | 323 |
| 66 | Obstetrics & Gynecology | 284 |
| 271 | X-ray | 13 |
| 168 | Orthopedics | 2 |
| 2,419 | Total Hours for Degree | 2,047 |

“*Chiropractic care optimizes whatever genetic abilities an individual has to resist disease.*”

–Ronald Pero

spoiler alert

*If you think chiropractic is just for back pain,*

consider

*that it can affect your overall health.*

Most people go to chiropractors because they have some type of back pain. It is true chiropractic helps back pain. However, chiropractors are much more than back doctors. They are first and foremost nervous system doctors. With spinal adjustments, the entire brain and nervous system are impacted. The spine is the "container to the nervous system." If there are blockages, meaning not all joints are moving correctly, there can be an impact on the brain, nerves, muscles, and organs that the nerves supply. If the blockages are cleared and the messages in the nervous system can flow freely, it will impact the health of not only the spine, but the health of your arms, legs, muscles, and organs.

Most people wait until they experience unbearable pain to see the chiropractor. Instead of being proactive, they embrace reactivity. Pain is often a signal that something is going on, but it doesn't often affect only at a spinal level. Most people stop going to the chiropractor when they are out of pain. Maybe they forget or maybe they don't know that a visit to the chiropractor can be a wellness experience. Chiropractors can give great insights into nutrition, exercise, stress strategies, and ways to help reverse the effects of the aging process and boost the immune system.

> "*Going to a chiropractor just for pain relief is like robbing a bank and only taking the pens.*"
>
> – Keith Wassung

## Fresh Ideas to Extend Your Expiration Date

Having a chiropractor who can address your lifestyle needs and health is essential for being well and staying well. Great chiropractors are a wealth of information with deep insight into how the body works. Start thinking of your chiropractor as a wellness professional. As with any profession, there are good ones and great ones. Find great ones by asking others whom they like, or if you are moving, ask your chiropractor to recommend someone in another city.

## Learn More

*The Power of Self-Healing: Unlock Your Natural Healing Potential in 21 Days!*, by Fabrizio Mancini, is an inspiring view of chiropractic, which includes helpful self-care tips.

*"The more mechanically distorted a person is, the less energy is available for thinking, metabolism, and healing."*

– Dr. Roger Sperry, Nobel Laureate

spoiler alert

*If you think chiropractic care is just for adults,*

consider

*that children and babies have a spine and nervous system, too.*

A common misconception about chiropractic care is that it is just for adults with back pain. Babies and children greatly benefit from chiropractic care, too, and they respond quickly because they don't have a long lifetime of poor spinal patterns. Their nervous systems and spines are generally very fluid and responsive.

In a study by G. Gutmann, it was estimated that 80 percent of newborns had some sort of nerve dysfunction at birth. Chiropractors are trained to address and adjust spinal misalignments that often result in nerve dysfunction. The nervous system controls the development of infants as they grow from infants to toddlers and into children and young adults. This is why any blocks in the nervous system are so vital to remove, so your children can grow up with the best possible expression of their nervous system.

Everyone benefits from having their nervous system function at 100 percent. How do you know if a child or baby needs to have his or her spine checked? For children, notice if they have had any falls, head bumps, or consistently struggle with coughs, colds, and ear aches. For babies, consider the birth process. In many cases, this is a traumatic experience with effects from the extreme force on the spine (especially the cervical spine/neck) from pulling, forceps, or vacuum extraction.

> “*The nervous system controls and coordinates all of the organs and structures of the human body.*” ”
>
> – *Gray's Anatomy*

## Fresh Ideas to Extend Your Expiration Date

Chiropractic is safe and effective for babies and children, although they may not have back pain. They often benefit from chiropractic care with improved posture, concentration, and an enhanced immune system. They are typically given light force, spinal adjustments with no pain or discomfort. As with anything, pick a chiropractor with a good reputation and experience adjusting children.

## Learn More

Two websites with information on how and why kids should be adjusted are icpa4kids.org and welladjusted.me.

A holistic, parenting resource is *Well Adjusted Babies: Your Complete Guide to Pregnancy, Birth, Babies, and Beyond*, by Jennifer Barham-Floreani.

# appendix

## Beverages

| WATER | | |
|---|---|---|
| **Savor These** | | **Avoid These** |
| • Filtered tap water<br>• Water from natural springs<br>• Water flavored with real mint, lemons, limes, oranges, etc.<br>• Water flavored with essential oils | **VERSUS** | • Bottled water (unless traveling in other countries)<br>• Unfiltered tap water<br>• Vitamin Water (33 grams of sugar per bottle)<br>• Zero-calorie, flavored waters<br>• Sports drinks (sugar-filled)<br>• Powdered water flavors<br>• Sodas (including diet sodas) |

| FRUIT/VEGGIE DRINKS | | |
|---|---|---|
| **Savor These** | | **Avoid These** |
| • Freshly made, mostly veggie smoothies<br>• Homemade juices (on occasion) | **VERSUS** | • Bottled smoothies: Naked, Odwalla, etc.<br>• Juice from concentrate (high-sugar content, no fiber to slow insulin spike) |

| TEA | | |
|---|---|---|
| **Savor These** | | **Avoid These** |
| • Unsweetened herbal teas | **VERSUS** | • Sweetened teas from Lipton, Snapple, etc. |

| CAFFEINATED BEVERAGES (USE SPARINGLY) | | |
|---|---|---|
| **Savor These** | | **Avoid These** |
| • Black tea<br>• Green tea<br>• Coffee with minimal sweeteners and full-fat cream or milk | **VERSUS** | • Energy drinks: Red Bull, Monster, etc.<br>• Energy shots<br>• Bottled coffees<br>• Store-bought flavored creamers (contain trans fats and unpronounceable ingredients) |

## Animal Products

| MEAT | | |
|---|---|---|
| **Savor These** | | **Avoid These** |
| • Organic, grass-fed beef<br>• Free-range chicken<br>• Elk<br>• Venison<br>• Duck<br>• Deer<br>• Buffalo<br>• Lamb | **VERSUS** | • Conventionally raised animals (never an option) |

| FISH | | |
|---|---|---|
| **Savor These** | | **Avoid These** |
| • Wild | **VERSUS** | • Farmed-raised: high in Omega-6 (inflammatory), especially Tilapia and Atlantic salmon |

| DAIRY | | |
|---|---|---|
| **Savor These** | | **Avoid These** |
| • Goat milk<br>• Cultured raw is best: yogurt, kefir, cheese, and raw milk<br>• Organic dairy is second best<br>• Whole dairy products help to better absorb the fat-soluble vitamins, less toxic additives, more fullness<br>• Butter<br>• Cream | **VERSUS** | • Nonorganic<br>• Milk containing rGBH, a GMO growth hormone<br>• Fat-free and skim<br>• Margarine or butter substitutes<br>• Nondairy substitutes<br>• Flavored yogurts |

## Fruit and Vegetables

| FRUITS | | |
|---|---|---|
| **Savor These** | | **Avoid These** |
| • Buy organic and local if possible. Anything with a thick peel that can be removed is okay if inorganic. If eating the peel, try to go organic to decrease pesticide exposure. | **VERSUS** | • EWG's 2012 Dirty Dozen list for most pesticides (most to least): apples, peaches, strawberries, nectarines (imported), grapes, and blueberries (domestic) |

| DRIED FRUITS | | |
|---|---|---|
| **Savor These** | | **Avoid These** |
| • Organic<br>• Small amounts (high glycemic index) | **VERSUS** | • With sugar<br>• With preservatives<br>• With added sugars |

| VEGETABLES | | |
|---|---|---|
| **Savor These** | | **Avoid These** |
| • Anything with a removable skin can be eaten inorganically. If eating the skin, organic, fresh, and local are best. Don't forget sea vegetables, such as nori, wakeme, etc. | **VERSUS** | • EWG's 2012 Dirty Dozen list for most pesticides (most to least): celery, bell peppers, spinach, lettuce, cucumbers, potatoes, kale, and green beans |

| POTATOES | | |
|---|---|---|
| **Savor These** | | **Avoid These** |
| • Yams<br>• Sweet Potatoes | **VERSUS** | • White Potatoes |

## Sides

| NUTS | | |
|---|---|---|
| **Savor These** | | **Avoid These** |
| • Raw<br>• Nut butters (preferably organic): almond butter and cashew butter | **VERSUS** | • Salted<br>• Roasted<br>• Peanuts (technically a legume) |

| SOY | | |
|---|---|---|
| **Savor These** | | **Avoid These** |
| • Fermented Soy<br>• Natto<br>• Tempeh<br>• Miso | **VERSUS** | • Processed soy products<br>• Tofu<br>• Soy sauce<br>• Edamame<br>• Soybeans<br>• Soy oil |

| BEANS | | |
|---|---|---|
| **Savor These** | | **Avoid These** |
| • Sprouted legumes/beans: can be inflammatory if not soaked and sprouted | **VERSUS** | • Unsprouted beans: difficult to digest, high on the glycemic index |

| GRAINS | | |
|---|---|---|
| **Savor These** | | **Avoid These** |
| • Sprouted grains only | **VERSUS** | • Completely eliminate all white grains.<br>• Limit or restrict all grains unless sprouted: includes white flour, wheat flour, whole grains, corn, oats, soy, barley, millet, rye, alfalfa, etc. |

| RICE | | |
|---|---|---|
| **Savor These** | | **Avoid These** |
| • Wild rice<br>• Brown rice (small amounts) | **VERSUS** | • White rice<br>• Puffed rice |

| DESSERTS | | |
|---|---|---|
| **Savor These** | | **Avoid These** |
| • Dark chocolate<br>• Fruit-based desserts or ice creams with no added sweeteners | **VERSUS** | • Cake mixes<br>• Brownie mixes<br>• Candy<br>• Store-bought ice cream<br>• Frozen desserts |

## Flavorings

| SWEET | | |
|---|---|---|
| **Savor These** | | **Avoid These** |
| • Small amounts of stevia<br>• High-quality grade maple syrup<br>• Local, raw honey | **VERSUS** | • Artificial sweeteners: aspartame, NutraSweet, Equal, neotame, sucralose, Splenda, saccharin, and SweetN' Low<br>• Agave nectar |

| SAVORY | | |
|---|---|---|
| **Savor These** | | **Avoid These** |
| • Herbs and spices (easy to grow and easy to dry): organic is best. Buy in bulk to save money and have readily available. | **VERSUS** | • Not adding fresh spices (won't reap benefits of enhanced taste and anti-inflammatory properties) |

| FATS | | |
|---|---|---|
| **Savor These** | | **Avoid These** |
| • peanut oil (in moderation)<br>• sesame oil (in moderation)<br>• extra virgin olive oil<br>• macadamia nut oil<br>• coconut oil: unrefined or virgin is the best<br>• fish oils<br>• walnut oil<br>• hemp oil<br>• flax seed oil (always use cold and refrigerate)<br>• palm oil<br>• animal fats from pastured or organic animals<br>• butter or ghee<br>• full-fat dairy products: raw and organic are best<br>• avocados<br>• olives<br>• nuts and nut butters, excluding peanuts (technically a legume)<br>• egg yolks | **VERSUS** | • canola oil<br>• soy or soybean oil<br>• sunflower oil<br>• cottonseed oil<br>• corn oil<br>• grape-seed oil<br>• low-fat or nonfat dairy products<br>• safflower oil<br>• margarine<br>• shortening<br>• hydrogenated and partially hydrogenated oils<br>• fats found in most non-butter spreads or salad dressings |

Your best health steps may be buying foods without labels and only eating foods that you know exactly what the constituents are.

- If this is not possible, then avoid products with ingredient labels that list artificial colorings, preservatives, natural flavors, light, diet, heart healthy, low fat, zero calories, low sugar, or no sugar.
- Avoid products with seals of approval from various organizations or with health claims.

- Avoid any foods that are white or can have white within them (e.g., bread, pasta, rice, and cereal).
- Try to eliminate microwaveable dinners, canned soups, canned food products (due to BPA*), most foods that come out of a box, and store-bought salad dressings.
- Avoid eating things that will never mold. If it doesn't naturally decompose, it may be difficult on your body to process.
- Stay away from fried foods, fast foods, and most anything found in a convenience store, except possibly for the fruit.
- Reduce exposure to Genetically Modified Products or GMO: soy, corn, canola, zucchini, yellow squash, sugar from sugar beets, and papaya. It is highly likely that these foods are genetically modified unless specifically labeled organic or GMO free.

*BPA, or Bisphenol A, is an endocrine disruptor that can mimic estrogen. It is shown to affect the thyroid and may contribute to certain types of cancers. It is also found in the lining of most canned goods. Unless they specifically state that they are BPA free, you can assume the cans contain BPA.

**Supplementation to Consider**. It is best to get your nutrients from whole foods, herbs, and spices. Here are four vitamins I personally recommend to my patients:

1. Multivitamins. This is simply because farmland and the fruit and veggies it produces are not as nutrient dense as they used to be.

2. Vitamin $D_3$. Entire books have been written on how deficient most people are in this vitamin. The bottom line is, you generally don't get enough sun exposure and rarely get sufficient amounts from your food.

3. Quality Omega-3 fatty acid. Omega-3 is essential, which means your body cannot manufacture it on its own. It is important to choose a high-quality Omega-3. Otherwise, it can easily oxidize, create free radicals, and lead to inflammation. This will hurt rather than help.

4. Probiotics. They help to rebalance intestinal bacteria, which easily becomes imbalanced with antibiotics, stress, and dietary factors. I personally recommend a liquid form with a variety of strains.

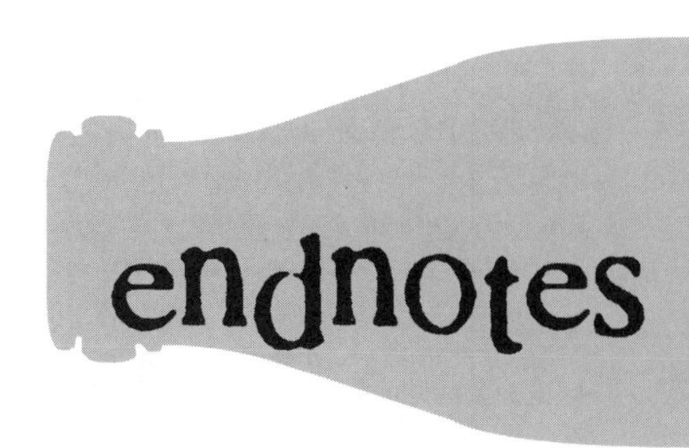


## Wellness

1. "Health, United States, 2010: With Special Feature on Death and Dying," *National Center for Health Statistics*, 2011, 2, http://www.cdc.gov/nchs/data/hus/hus10.pdf.

## Food

1. Crystal Smith-Spangler et al., "Are Organic Foods Safer or Healthier Than Conventional Alternatives? A Systematic Review," Annals of Internal Medicine, September 2012, 157, no. 5, 348–366.
2. A. Velimirov, C. Binter, and J. Zentek, "Biological Effects of Transgenic Maize NK603xMON810 Fed in Long-Term Reproduction Studies in Mice," *Federal Ministry of Health, Family, and Youth*, 2008, http://annals.org/article.aspx?articleid=1355685.
3. J. S. de Vendomois et al., "A Comparison of the Effects of Three GM Corn Varieties on Mammalian Health," *International Journal of Biological Sciences* 5, no. 7 (2009): 706–726, doi:10.7150/ijbs.5.706.
4. G. E. Séralini et al., "Long Term Toxicity of a Roundup Herbicide and a Roundup-Tolerant Genetically Modified Maize," *Food and Chemical Toxicology*, 2012, 50, no. 11, http://dx.doi.org/10.1016/j.fct.2012.08.005.
5. Yang Qing, "Gain Weight by Going Diet? Artificial Sweeteners and the Neurobiology of Sugar Cravings," *Yale Journal of Biology and Medicine*, June 2010, 83, no. 2, 101–108, http://www.ncbi.nlm.nih.gov/pmc/issues/188074/.
6. Selin, Bolca et al., "Disposition of Soy Isoflavones in Normal Human Breast Tissue," *American Journal of Clinical Nutrition* 91, no. 4 (April 2010): 976–984, doi:10.3945 /ajcn.2009.28854.

7. Hal Herzog, "Why Do Most Vegetarians Go Back to Eating Meat?," *Psychology Today*, June 20, 2011, http://www.psychologytoday.com/blog/animals-and-us/201106/why-do-most-vegetarians-go-back-eating-meat.
8. Thomas Jefferson, "Dinner is Served," *Thomas Jefferson's Monticello*, May 1, 2008, http://www.monticello.org/site/jefferson/dinner-served.
9. Amy Joy Lanou, "Bone Health in Children: Guidelines for Calcium Intake Should Be Revised," *British Medical Journal* 333, no. 7572 (October 2006): 763–764, doi:10.1136/bmj.38996.499410.BE.
10. "Food, Nutrition, Physical Activity, and the Prevention of Cancer: A Global Perspective," *World Cancer Research Fund, American Institute for Cancer Research*, (Washington, DC: AICR, 2007), http://www.hsph.harvard.edu/nutritionsource/what-should-you-eat/calcium-full-story/index.html.
11. J. M. Genkinger et al., "Dairy Products and Ovarian Cancer: A Pooled Analysis of 12 Cohort Studies," *Cancer Epidemiology, Biomarkers, and Prevention*, 2006, 15, 364–72, http://www.ncbi.nlm.nih.gov/pubmed/16492930?dopt=Citation.

## Movement

1. Arthur C. Guyton and John E. Hall, *Textbook of Medical Physiology*, 11th Edition (Philadelphia: Saunders, 2005), 1055.
2. "Thin People Can Be Fat on the Inside," *Associated Press*, May 11, 2007, http://www.msnbc.msn.com/id/18594089/ns/health-fitness/t/thin-people-can-be-fat-inside/#.UA4MKGFWqSo.
3. Gretchen Reynolds, *The First 20 Minutes: Surprising Science Reveals How We Can; Exercise Better, Train Smarter, Live Longer* (New York: Hudson Street Press, 2012), 194.

## Emotions

1. Robert Emery and Jim Coan, "What Causes Chest Pain When Feelings Are Hurt?," *Scientific American*, February 19, 2010, http://www.scientificamerican.com/article.cfm?id=what-causes-chest-pains.
2. Susan K. Urahn et al., "Pursuing the American Dream Economic Mobility across Generations," July 2012, http://www.pewtrusts.org/uploadedFiles/wwwpewtrustsorg/Reports/Economic_Mobility/Pursuing_American_Dream.pdf.
3. Branko Milanovic, *The Haves and the Have-Nots: A Brief and Idiosyncratic History of Global Inequality* (New York: Basic Books, 2012), 116.

## Chemical Peer Pressure

1. "Children and Chemicals," *Mount Sinai Hospital*, accessed September 16, 2012, http://www.mountsinai.org/patient-care/service-areas/children/areas-of-care /childrens-environmental-health-center/overview/children-and-chemicals.
2. Halina Szejnwald Brown, Donna Bishop, and Carol Rowan, "The Role of Skin Absorption as a Route of Exposure for Volatile Organic Compounds (VOCs) in Drinking Water," *American Journal of Public Health*, 1984, 74, no. 5, http://ajph.aphapublications.org/doi /pdf/10.2105/AJPH.74.5.479.
3. C. F. Garland et al., "Vitamin D and Prevention of Breast Cancer: Pooled Analysis," *Journal of Steroid Biochemistry and Molecular Biology* 103, nos. 3–5 (March 2007): 708–11.
4. E. D. Gorham et al., "Optimal Vitamin D Status for Colorectal Cancer Prevention: A Quantitative Meta-analysis," *American Journal of Preventative Medicine*, March 2007, 32, no. 3, 210–16.
5. "Prescribing Information for Flulaval," accessed August 21, 2012, http://www.fda.gov /downloads/BiologicsBloodVaccines/Vaccines/ApprovedProducts/ucm112904.pdf.
6. "Flu Vaccine Effectiveness: Questions and Answers for Health Professionals," *Centers for Disease Control*, last modified October 12, 2011, http://www.cdc.gov/flu/professionals /vaccination/effectivenessqa.htm.
7. Lorna Benson, "Flu Vaccine Not as Effective as Thought, New Study Says," *Minnesota Public Radio*, last modified October 25, 2011, http://minnesota.publicradio.org/display /web/2011/10/25/university-of-minnesota-flu-vaccine-study/.
8. Michael T. Osterholm et al., "Efficacy and Effectiveness of Influenza Vaccines: A Systematic Review and Meta-analysis," *The Lancet Infectious Diseases* 12, no. 1 (January 1, 2012): 36–44, doi:10.1016/S1473-3099(11)70295-X.
9. K. K. Cheng, Iain Chalmers, and Trevor A. Sheldon, "Adding Fluoride to Water Supplies," *British Medical Journal* 335, no. 7622 (October 6, 2007): 699–702, doi:10.1136/bmj .39318.562951.BE.
10. "Community Water Fluoridation," *Centers for Disease Control*, last modified June 18, 2012, http://www.cdc.gov/fluoridation/fact_sheets/engineering/wfadditives.htm.
11. W. Mundy et al., "Building a Database of Developmental Neurotoxicants: Evidence from Human and Animal Studies," accessed October 1, 2012, http://www.epa.gov/ncct /toxcast/files/summit/48P%20Mundy%20TDAS.pdf.

12. Charles Duhig, "U. S. Bolsters Chemical Restrictions for Water," *The New York Times*, last modified March 22, 2010, http://www.nytimes.com/2010/03/23/business/23water.html.
13. "Reinvigorated Bottled Water Bounces Back from Recessionary Years: New Report from Beverage Marketing Corporation Shows Volume Reaches a New High Point," *Beverage Marketing Corporation*, May 2012, http://beveragemarketing.com/?section=pressreleases.
14. Charles Fishman, "U.S. Bottled Water Sales Are Booming (Again) Despite Opposition," *National Geographic*, last modified May 17, 2012, http://newswatch.nationalgeographic.com/2012/05/17/u-s-bottled-water-sales-are-booming-again-despite-opposition/.

## Popular Health Beliefs

1. Ross DeVol et al., "An Unhealthy America: The Economic Burden of Chronic Disease—Charting a New Course to Save Lives and Increase Productivity and Economic Growth," October 2007, http://www.milkeninstitute.org/publications/publications.taf?function=detail&ID=38801018
2. H. C. Kung et al., "Deaths: Final Data for 2005," *National Vital Statistics Reports* 2008, 56, http://www.cdc.gov/nchs/data/nvsr/nvsr56/nvsr56_10.pdf.
3. Mary J. Renfrew et al., "Preventing Disease and Saving Resources: The Potential Contribution of Increasing Breastfeeding Rates in the U. K.," October 2012, 7, http://www.unicef.org.uk/Documents/Baby_Friendly/Research/Preventing_disease_saving_resources.pdf?epslanguage=en.
4. Samantha Shapiro, "Mommy Wars: The Prequel Ina May Gaskin and the Battle for At-Home Births," *The New York Times*, May 23, 2012, http://www.nytimes.com/2012/05/27/magazine/ina-may-gaskin-and-the-battle-for-at-home-births.html
5. Judith Lothian, "Home Birth: The Wave of the Future?," *The Journal of Perinatal Education*, Summer 2006, 15, no. 3, http://www.ncbi.nlm.nih.gov/pmc/articles/PMC1595304/.

# acknowledgments

I am extraordinarily grateful to many wonderful people who helped this book become tangible.

First, to Maryanna Young at Aloha Publishing, for suggesting that I write a book and assisting me in developing the concepts behind it. I would not and could not have done this without you. Thank you for helping me navigate this uncharted territory into my first book.

Cover designer Cari Campbell, for far surpassing my imagination; Shiloh Schroeder, for the interior; and Kim Foster, for editing.

I am grateful to Dr. Dustin Thomas for inspiring me to join the chiropractic profession. Colleagues and staff at Live Right Chiropractic: Dr. Yvonne Honovich, Dr. Michelle Fisher, Jessica, Joan, and Tish. You literally watched me write it and didn't seem to get too tired of hearing about it.

To the Summer Authors' group: Michele, Joel, Brandon, Kelly, Rob, and Hannah. Your weekly support and camaraderie made this a great experience.

I am grateful to the support of my friends, Heather and Matt, for being a sounding board for concepts. To Crystal, for a long afternoon of driving and creativity and to Dr. Laine Morales, for enriching my life and being awesome.

Bompa and Nana, thanks for being my biggest fans and cheerleaders.

To my family who witnessed this process from afar and offered insight when they could: Mom, Dad, Grandma. To Janette, Sarah, Liz, and Gabby—I love you more than you can imagine.

To Chip, thanks for the support, leaving me alone when I needed it, and most of all for understanding. Thanks for not getting too frustrated when I would say, "I can't talk, clean, travel…I need to write."

# about the author

**Dr. Angela Young** is passionate about helping you get well and stay well. She gives you the resources you will need to make great lifetime decisions for you and your family. She holds a Bachelor of Science in Health and Wellness and a Doctor of Chiropractic degree from Parker University. She is a Registered Yoga Teacher (RYT 200), bringing all of her education together into perfect harmony and balance. For more information, visit angelayoungdc.com.